PRACTISE WHAT YOU PREACH

By the same author

PRACTICE MAKES PERFECT

PRACTISE WHAT YOU PREACH

Edward Vernon

ISBN 0 333 24309 9

First published 1978 by
MACMILLAN LONDON LIMITED
4 Little Essex Street London WC2R 3LF
and Basingstoke
Associated Companies in Delhi, Dublin,
Hong Kong, Johannesburg, Lagos, Melbourne,
New York, Singapore and Tokyo

Printed in Great Britain by
THE ANCHOR PRESS LTD
Tiptree, Essex
Bound in Great Britain by
WM BRENDON AND SON LTD
Tiptree, Essex

To Helen and Neil.
Special thanks to Peter Collenette.

E.V.

I

AT FOUR O'CLOCK IN THE MORNING I got up from Mrs Suggett's lumpy double bed, pulled on my raincoat and set off for home. With a little luck, I thought, I might be able to slip into my own bed without waking my wife. We had been married a week and Margaret had still not got used to the fact that I would sometimes go to bed five or six times a night. She was new to the world where husbands spend the night flitting from bedroom to bedroom.

Mrs Suggett had just delivered her fifth child, firing the infant from her womb with experienced ease. The midwife, Miss Wilde, had been standing in a close catching position but had been momentarily distracted by Mr Suggett, who had been celebrating prematurely with a litre bottle of expensive malt whisky, and who had been anxious to share his celebration with another. Miss Wilde had been the only available drinking companion, and consequently when Mrs Suggett's fifth was making its way into the world the hands which should have directed its journey were occupied instead with a half-pint glass containing a generous measure of alcohol.

As a result of this lapse Mrs Suggett had suffered a small tear, which required suturing. All of which explains how I came to be pulling my raincoat on in her bedroom.

It had been one of those nights that general practitioners dread. The telephone had rung for the first time just as I was taking off my trousers a few minutes before midnight.

'Can you come out?' the caller enquired.

'What's the trouble?' I asked, hopping on one leg while trying to decide whether to take my trousers off completely or put them back on again.

'It's our mam,' said the voice at the other end.

'What's wrong with your mam?' Telephone tucked under

my ear, I reached for the pen in my jacket pocket. The jacket was already hanging in the wardrobe, and I could just reach it.

'She's bad,' answered the caller.

'Any particular kind of bad?' I asked. I decided to take off my trousers anyway and stand on both legs.

'I don't know,' replied the voice.

Just then Margaret came into the bedroom and absent-mindedly switched off the light. As a result I was left standing in the dark on one leg, with the telephone in my right hand and my left hand inside my jacket pocket hunting for a pen. Naturally I fell over.

'What's the address?' I screamed into the telephone as I crashed on to the floor.

'Flat 6, Fowler Mansions, Ball Street,' answered the caller immediately.

'Put the light on,' I cried. I couldn't move as my trousers were wrapped tightly around my ankles.

'Pardon?' said the voice at the other end.

'Put the light on,' I said, with unusual presence of mind, 'then I'll be able to find the flat quickly.'

'I would,' he replied, 'if I could.'

I hung up, muttering the address to myself.

'What are you doing?' asked Margaret calmly. She had switched the light on again.

'Flat 6, Fowler Mansions, Ball Street,' I called to her. 'Write it down.'

'You'll ruin those trousers,' said Margaret, picking up a note-pad and pencil from the bedside table where they'd been hiding behind the telephone.

I dressed silently, slowly and carefully, tore the address from the top of the notepad, and kissed her. Then I made my way downstairs. In the car I switched on the interior light, opened my street-map, and examined the piece of notepaper. 'Two pints today, please,' it said. I got out of the car and made my way back upstairs again.

'I put the address in your jacket pocket while you got dressed,' explained Margaret. 'Hurry back,' she added, blowing me a kiss as I headed for the stairs again.

Outside it was raining hard. The moon was as slim and use-less as a nail-paring, and the only light came from the streetlamps. Ball Street is on the other side of the town in an area carefully described by relatively honest estate agents as 'convenient for the railway station'. Most of the houses were built a century or so ago and were once occupied by wealthy families and their servants. Today they are divided into flats and the only servants in residence are civil.

Even inexperienced general practitioners soon develop the knack of reading house-numbers on dark wet nights while driving by at thirty miles an hour. I wound my window down and stuck my head out in the rain to get a better view. The original residents of Ball Street had been too smart to give their homes numbers. The houses all had names.

It took me ten minutes of patient work to find Fowler Mansions, another five to spot the front door of Flat 6, and a further ten to discover that it could only be approached from the rear up what had been a fire-escape. When I finally hammered on the door I was drenched.

'Here's the doc, Mam,' called the youth who opened the door. 'I told you I'd rung,' he sniffed defiantly.

'We thought you wasn't coming,' complained a middle-aged man in an off-white vest and dark-blue trousers.

'Hullo, Doc,' called a voice from well inside the room. It was too dark to see its owner, but I recognised it as belonging to Mrs Temple, a regular visitor to the surgery.

I started gingerly towards it.

'Have you got a light?' I asked.

'Sure,' said the man in the vest. 'Have one of mine.' He generously thrust a packet of cigarettes into my face.

'No,' I said. 'I meant is there a light in the room?'

'The Electricity Board have cut us off,' said Mrs Temple sadly.

'They said we owed them money,' the man complained as though innocent and rather bewildered by their action.

Slowly my eyes got used to the darkness and I could see the dim outline of Mrs Temple. I put down my black bag and sat on the edge of the bed. She smiled at me, and I reached out for where I thought her hand should be.

Taking the patient's pulse does not always provide a great deal in the way of useful information but it does break the ice and give the inexperienced doctor a few quiet moments in which to make a preliminary assessment. Sit as if concentrating and counting and most patients will keep still and quiet. Besides, I always feel that it is slightly improper to thrust one's finger into a patient's most private cavities without first observing conventional social mores. Taking a patient's pulse is a sort of professional greeting.

When I reached for Mrs Temple's hand I was expecting to feel an ordinary fleshy hand, the type you'd see hanging on the end of almost any arm. I didn't expect to find myself clutching a slender hairy paw ending in thin sharp nails. My alarm must have shown.

'Let me move the dog, Doc,' said Mr Temple, leaning across me and lashing out in the gloom with a newspaper. An enormous dark beast leapt off Mrs Temple and brushed past me. My heart, which had already stopped, was so surprised that it started again. I wondered if my hair had turned grey or gone straight to white.

'What's been the trouble?' I asked Mrs Temple when I'd recovered my composure.

'It's my head,' came the reply.

'What's been the trouble with it?'

'It hurts,' she said.

'You've got a headache?' I enquired.

'That's right.'

'Whereabouts?'

'In my head,' she answered neatly.

'Do you want a cup of coffee, Doctor?' asked Mr Temple. 'We've got a gas-ring.'

'I mean whereabouts in your head,' I explained to his wife after declining his offer.

'Oh, in the back,' she said.

I remembered then that she had for several years been under treatment for high blood-pressure. I couldn't recall the name or the dosage of the drug she was taking.

'Have you got your pills?' I asked her.

'They're in the cupboard, Doctor,' said Mrs Temple. She told the youth who'd telephoned to show them to me, and I followed him across the room to a small cupboard above a large cracked white sink.

The cupboard had three shelves each about eighteen inches

long and nine inches deep. Each shelf was packed tightly with bottles of pills. Most of the bottles were still full.

'What's all this?' I called to Mrs Temple.

'My pills.'

'But they're supposed to be in you, not in the cupboard.'

'They don't agree with me, Doctor,' she said. 'I go all dizzy when I take them.'

'How many years have you been putting pills in here?' I asked.

'Four or five,' she replied. 'Ever since Dr Oaks started me off on them.'

'Why didn't you say they didn't suit you?' I asked her.

'I didn't want to upset anyone,' she replied.

I opened my bag and extracted my sphygmomanometer, intending to take her blood-pressure. It was so dark, however, that I couldn't see the dial. I decided to concede victory to the Electricity Board.

'I'm going to send you into hospital,' I told her. 'I can't examine you properly here.'

Her son led me down the fire-escape and across the road to the nearest public telephone. We waited outside in the rain while a pair of giggling teenaged girls enjoyed a long and obviously stimulating conversation with a talkative someone somewhere. When they eventually emerged I called an ambulance and arranged with the local hospital for the house physician to have a bed ready for Mrs Temple. Then I went back to the flat with her son and told her what I had arranged.

'That's very good of you, Doctor,' she said. 'But I didn't expect you to get me into hospital.'

'I bet they'll have telly on the ward,' said Mr Temple with undisguised envy.

'I really just wanted you to have a look at my head,' Mrs Temple said. 'Just to make sure I hadn't broken anything.'

'Broken anything?'

'Where I hit it when I tripped over the dog,' she explained. 'It's dark in here,' she added rather unnecessarily.

'You didn't have a headache until then?'

She shook the object of our deliberations.

With this new history in mind I examined her skull. There were no signs of any broken bones or broken skin.

'I thought perhaps you'd have a couple of aspirin tablets you could give me,' she said.

'You'd better come along to the surgery tomorrow,' I told her, 'so I can check your blood-pressure.'

She said she would. I gave her two aspirin tablets and hurried back down the fire-escape towards the telephone, hoping to stop the ambulance setting out. I was too late. Before I had even picked up the receiver it pulled up outside Fowler Mansions with an impressive array of blue and orange emergency-lamps lighting up the wet pavements. It took me five minutes to persuade the men to return to their depot without a patient.

When I got home there was a note on my pillow from Margaret asking me to go and see Mrs Suggett at Flat 4, Fowler Mansions, Ball Street. She told me later that she'd had great difficulty in persuading the two girls who'd rung to stop giggling and give her the correct address.

2

IT HAD BEEN RAINING NON-STOP for a week. The drains and
gutters in Hungerford Road had long since given up trying to
cope with the deluge. At one spot near the corner of Codnip
Terrace the roadway had turned into a small lake. As I pulled
up outside the surgery after spending the small hours recon-
structing Mrs Suggett's battered perineal architecture the clouds
received reinforcements and the seven-day shower became a
violent storm.

Sitting in the car and waiting for the rain to subside a little
so that I could make my way into the house without getting
drenched again, I peered out through the raindrop-speckled
windows at the shadowy lines of the surgery. Built a century
before as a private house, it was sturdy, double-fronted and
handsome in a rugged sort of way. To its right lay the garage,
once a stable, which was approached by a drive consisting of
equal parts of weed and gravel. The front door, situated in the
centre of the house between two huge bay windows, was
approached by a straight crazy-paving path dividing the front
garden into two more or less equal halves. On both sides there
were lawns, and in the centre of each lawn a circular island
rose-bed. I sat, parked in the road since the journey from there
to the front door was slightly less puddly and hazardous than
the journey from the drive to front door, and waited for the
storm to let up.

When Dr Oaks had decided to retire he had offered to sell me
the house and surgery.

'I'm going to find a little cottage in the country,' he told me,
'have the doorbell and telephone disconnected and live a silent
life.' Silence, it seemed, was the luxury he craved more than
any other.

He had arranged for a local estate agent to value the property, and at my request the manager of the local branch of a national building society had generously agreed to make the necessary loan.

'I shan't want much of the furniture,' Dr Oaks told me. 'You can have what you want when I've moved the stuff I'm taking with me. It's a wedding present.'

Since the only furniture Margaret and I possessed was a portable record-player and a folding card-table we were grateful. The house had eleven good-sized rooms in all and, even with the most vivid imagination in the world, it is difficult to make a house that size look anything like occupied with only a portable record-player and a folding card-table. There are bound to be gaps.

Dr Oaks moved out just after Christmas, and Margaret and I moved in just before the New Year. Since neither she nor I had wanted speeches or fuss we'd married quietly in a register office in a town a few miles away where no one knew either of us. The ceremony was over by lunchtime, and that same afternoon we collected the key to my surgery and our home.

At the front of the house, on the left as you looked from the road, was the waiting-room. Net curtains protected the patients within from public view. The surgery was at the back of the house, looking on to the back garden. Once seen, patients would pass through the french windows, follow the pathway round to the side of the house, and leave through the garage.

The other front bay window belonged to the sitting-room, which was traditionally kept for the doctor's private use. Dr Oaks had had a lock put on to its door after he had once discovered two small boys playing football with the magnificent globe of the world which, when unmolested, perched proudly on a wooden stand near the window.

Behind the sitting-room were the dining-room and the kitchen. Upstairs, Dr Oaks had divided off a small flat, which had at one time been occupied by a housekeeper but was later my home for a while when I worked as his assistant. Apart from the flat there was a master bedroom and bathroom and a spare bedroom, all more or less empty of loose furniture, although Margaret and I had moved an old bed and rickety bedside table from the flat into the master bedroom at the front of the house.

Besides the furniture which Dr Oaks had given us I had purchased most of his equipment from him. There were the chairs and table in the waiting-room, the horsehair examination-couch, the battered leather-topped desk and chairs in the surgery and the metal filing-cabinets in which the patients' notes were stored. Dr Oaks had insisted on keeping his own stethoscope as a souvenir, but the rest of the paraphernalia which had filled the surgery's cupboards and drawers he had bequeathed to me.

It took me a day and a half to sort it out. Obsessed by curiosity, I counted eighty-seven sheets of blotting-paper in various stages of use and misuse, some virginal, some irretrievably ink-sodden. There were over one hundred pens which had at one time or another been donated by drug company representatives and which had ended their working lives years before. Oddly enough, they were all ballpoint and should have rendered the blotting-paper superfluous. Most of them carried advertisements for pharmaceutical products which had long ago been abandoned as too dangerous, too cheap or too old-fashioned. In a drawer at the bottom of the desk I found a forgotten box of thalidomide tablets, the various parts of an ear-syringe which had been taken apart and never put back together again, and a heap of old batteries of many shapes and sizes. Dr Oaks was a hoarder.

Slowly the rain began to ease off. I buttoned up my raincoat, pulled my ancient fishing-hat down over my ears and leapt out of the car. Inevitably I dropped the keys as I fumbled to lock it and, by the time I'd retrieved them, opened the gate and sprinted up the path to the front door, I was soaking wet. In the hall I hung my raincoat on one of the long row of empty pegs which would be festooned with patients' hats, scarves, coats and umbrellas in a few hours' time. I kicked off my shoes and wearily climbed up the stairs, making a mental note as I went to ask my secretary Miss Williams to telephone the man who was supposed to be making the brass plate for the front door and get him to hurry up. The space left by the removal of Dr Oaks' plate cried out to be filled.

Upstairs in our bedroom Margaret was fast asleep. I tiptoed in, using my pocket torch to light the way to the bed. I'd moved hardly more than a foot into the room when there was a crashing and clattering that would have awakened a hibernating tortoise. I fumbled for the switch and turned on the light. Behind the door lay half a dozen saucepans.

Margaret sat up in bed pointing a rolling-pin at my stomach.

'Don't move!' she screamed.

'It's me,' I shouted.

'Oh,' she sighed, putting her weapon down on the pillow and rubbing her eyes.

'That's the fourth time this week you've laid a booby trap for me,' I protested.

'Not for you,' she contradicted. 'It's in case we get burgled while you're out. I don't like sleeping on my own.'

'Well, if you want to lay booby traps, why not tell me what you're planning?' I said. I still bore scars from a collision, earlier in the week, with a galvanised bucket she had left in the middle of the floor.

'There's no point in setting the same trap every time,' said Margaret. 'Otherwise it wouldn't be a trap.'

I began to explain that it wasn't me she was trying to guard against; but by that time I'd got my clothes off and was lying in bed and, even at half-past four in the morning, there are better subjects for conversation than home-made burglar alarms when you've only been married a week.

Our alarm-clock has no finer feelings and no sense of compassion. It rang as usual at eight, and since we deliberately kept it on the window-sill I had to get out of bed to turn it off. I padded downstairs to put the kettle on and fetch the morning's mail; Margaret pulled on her dressing-gown and followed me.

When he had moved, Dr Oaks had arranged with the local post office to redirect mail addressed to him personally and had given us permission to open any letters addressed simply to 'The Doctor'. Apart from a handful of circulars and give-away medical magazines there were only three letters that morning. The first two I opened were from patients requesting repeat prescriptions. The third, posted two days previously, carried a simple if startling message. I read it twice before handing it to Margaret. This is what it said:

Dear Doctor,
Could you please call at no. 38 Barton Towers at your convenience. Mr Board has gone over.

Yours respectfully,
Alice Board (Mrs)

I copied down the name and address into the diary which I used to record my daily visits and began to attack the bowl of cereal which Margaret had put before me on the kitchen table.

It was two and a half hours later, after surgery, that I finally sat down in the car. Mr Board's was the first name on the list, and I drove round there in some trepidation. His wife was clearly one of those patients – all too rare, so some say – who regard the doctor's time as precious and hesitate to call him unnecessarily. Indeed, it might be said that inviting the doctor with so little sign of haste to certify death errs on the side of over-cautiousness.

I climbed the stairs at Barton Towers, my respect for Mrs Board's old-fashioned sense of propriety mixed with some dismay at the prospect before me. Even in cold wet weather the human body, its own heating system not in operation, is likely to fall into malodorous disrepair with indecent haste.

Mrs Board answered the front-door bell without delay, and to my relief there was no draught of death from within.

'I'm sorry to hear about Mr Board,' I said sympathetically.

'Oh yes,' she said, 'I'm sorry too.'

'It'll be a loss, of course,' I continued, 'but we have to go on.'

She seemed surprisingly unmoved by her husband's demise and puzzled by my clumsy expressions of sympathy.

'Is he in the bedroom?' I asked.

'He's out.'

'Out?' I repeated. 'They've taken him away, then?'

'No,' she said, puzzled. 'He's gone to work.'

'I thought . . .,' I stammered. 'You said he'd gone over. . . .'

'He has,' she said. 'He's gone over to Dr Edwards now that Dr Oaks has retired. But I'm staying with you. Can I have some more of my pills?'

She looked at me as if she were regretting her decision.

3

WE AWOKE NEXT MORNING to find that the rain had stopped at last. Miss Williams arrived as Margaret and I finished breakfast, and shortly afterwards the first patient wandered into the waiting-room. Before leaving the kitchen we peeped through the keyhole to see that the hall was clear. We had already learnt that if either of us ever tried to cross the hall while patients were *en route* to the waiting-room the results could be disastrous.

'I'm glad I caught you, Doctor,' the patient would beam. 'I didn't want to waste your time in the surgery with something so trivial, but I just wanted your advice about this.' So saying, he or she would remove a shoe and sock, pull up a trouser-leg or unbutton a jumper to expose the faulty item for examination. Meanwhile I would be hopping on one leg, desperate to reach the lavatory and get rid of the morning's first cup of coffee before surgery started, or, conscious of the fact that my chin was still smeared with cornflakes and marmalade, anxious to flee to the bathroom for a moment's privacy.

Nor would Margaret be able to escape.

'I'm glad I caught you, Mrs Vernon,' the patient would exclaim. 'I didn't want to waste the doctor's time, but I wanted to ask him about Trevor's little rash. That cream he gave us hasn't cleared it up yet and I wondered if I should try the stuff Dr Oaks gave Melinda last summer.' She was regularly asked about the best way to deal with a fractious cat having kittens, the type of milk to feed a colicky baby and the opening-times of the various chemists' shops.

Having successfully traversed the hall twice, I settled down in the surgery to begin the morning's work.

Mrs Hollins entered with a rush that left a quart glass bottle of thick, viscous cough medicine, inherited from Dr Oaks, smashed into countless pieces on the surgery floor.

'They say I can't look after David,' she said, when she'd finished apologising and I'd finished insisting that it mattered not at all.

'Who's David?' I asked her. 'And who says that you can't look after him?'

'Mrs Knott,' she said breathlessly. 'She's a child care officer.'

'And why does she say that?'

'David is Mrs Abberley's little boy,' she explained. 'She goes to work three mornings a week and I look after him.'

'How old is David?' I asked, by now thoroughly bewildered.

'Four.'

'But why does the child care officer say you can't look after him?' I asked her, when I'd finally worked out what she'd told me.

'I'm not properly certified,' she said unhappily. 'She says I have to be, to look after someone else's child.'

'Ah,' said I. The rules and regulations which direct the activities of social workers of all kinds never fail to confuse me.

'Can you do anything, Doctor?' she asked. She sat back, apparently drained of protest.

'I'm afraid not,' I admitted. 'If the social workers insist that you do not have the necessary certificate, then all I can suggest is that you ask them how best to get it.'

She left in obvious distress. She walked straight through the puddle of cough medicine, and her footsteps were clearly visible across the hall's parquet floor for several months, despite Margaret's strenuous efforts with scrubbing-brush and polish.

Although the patients a general practitioner sees usually seek advice as individuals, it is, of course, impossible to treat people in isolation. One man's chickenpox may be another man's shingles, and one woman's cold can be another patient's pneumonia. Even an apparently minor problem can have far-reaching effects on the lives of others. I had little idea just how much Mrs Hollins' lack of proper certification was about to influence the lives of other patients.

Evening surgery had been finished for over half an hour. For the third time that day I'd polished the new brass plate on the front door, and I was busily wolfing down the split-pea soup and peaches that Margaret had prepared for supper (to the casual reader our diet might seem a little odd, but we had inherited a number of old cans of food from Dr Oaks and for some inexplicable reason most of them were bare of labels; consequently meals were very largely a matter of chance) when the doorbell rang.

'Oh dear,' said Margaret.

'Oh damn,' said I.

'I thought you were off duty tonight.'

'I am.'

'I'll go and see who it is.'

'You wash up,' I said. 'I'll go.'

'Hullo,' grinned Dr Oaks as I gingerly opened the front door ready to make my excuses. 'Busy?'

'Not just at the moment,' I told him with a smile of relief. 'Come in. It's good to see you.'

'I've come to see if I can drag you off to a meeting,' he said. 'The local medical association is having its New Year clinical dinner.'

'What on earth is a clinical dinner?' I said.

'It's a dinner,' he explained, 'that is tax deductible. If we have some fellow to give us a lecture, the whole thing counts as a necessary part of our postgraduate education and the refreshments we need are partly paid for by the Chancellor, who is always eager to encourage us in our quest for enlightenment. I meant to let you know before, but circumstances prevented me.'

'Circumstances?' I echoed.

'I forgot,' he admitted.

'I don't know whether I can eat another meal,' I told him. 'Roast beef,' he said.

At that I led him into the kitchen and explained to Margaret that I'd been invited to attend a postgraduate lecture.

'What's it on?' asked Margaret.

'I haven't the foggiest,' he admitted. He reached into his coat pocket and produced three engraved tickets. 'I've got another spare, if you'd like to come,' he said to Margaret.

We drove in Dr Oaks' car. After a month's retirement his standard of driving had not improved. He still used the white lines in the centre of the road as a monorail train uses its rail, keeping two wheels on one side of it and two on the other in the comfortable knowledge that he would be unlikely to hit the kerb or collide with a parked car. Other vehicles in motion were expected to take the necessary avoiding action.

'It's about time you met some of your fellow-doctors in the town,' said Dr Oaks as we drove. 'Now that you're a fully fledged general practitioner you'll be expected to play your part in the medical life of the community.'

'Oh dear,' said Margaret. 'What does that involve?'

'Going to a clinical dinner every six months or so,' he replied.

'And?' I enquired.

'That's all,' he said. 'It isn't a particularly active medical community.'

'How many other doctors are there in the town?' I asked.

'About a dozen altogether,' he said. 'You know Dr Edwards, of course,' he went on, narrowly avoiding a Keep Left sign which had been carelessly abandoned in the middle of the road. 'He's been in general practice here for about thirty years and he and I always looked after each other's patients.'

'I made the same arrangement with him,' I said. 'I look after his on some nights and he looks after mine on the others.'

'And you've met Dr White, haven't you?' said Dr Oaks.

'The consultant physician?'

'That's right.'

'There's a Dr Williamson too,' I said. 'He's the medical officer at the cardboard-box factory, isn't he?'

'And a general practitioner,' nodded Dr Oaks, giving the driver of an oncoming bus a chance to test his coronary arteries. 'He's in practice with Dr Green and Dr Vance. They work mostly at the bottom end of the town.'

The meeting was being held in the dining-room of a hotel which usually catered for coachloads of foreign tourists, come to gaze at the numerous pieces of badly plumbed architectural heritage which are scattered throughout the local countryside. Dr Oaks parked – or, rather, stopped his car – right outside the hotel, ignoring the fact that the kerbside was already packed.

'Oh, thank you,' said Margaret. 'Are you dropping us off first?'

Dr Oaks looked at her in surprise. 'No,' he said.

'He's parked,' I whispered.

Margaret, not used to people leaving their cars double-parked in the darkness of a winter evening without lights, seemed to think I was joking. Only when Dr Oaks walked into the hotel with us did she realise that he was serious.

'Are you going to leave it unlocked?' she asked.

'Of course,' he said. 'If I lock it, how are the police going to move it?'

The hotel was having a busy evening. A blackboard announced that in one room a large car firm was holding a film show for its customers, while in the banqueting-hall there was a wedding reception. A scribbled and suitably indecipherable message at the bottom informed us that the doctors' dinner was being held in the Pink Suite on the third floor.

We struggled up the stairs. The lift seemed to be serving as an overflow room for the wedding guests.

Dr Oaks introduced us to most of the other diners. Two doctors were wearing dinner jackets, two dark suits, three sports jackets and slacks, and the rest tweed suits in varying stages of disrepair. The half-dozen ladies accompanying their husbands were wearing an equally mixed collection of clothes. Dr Edwards shook me warmly by the hand, Dr White remembered me, Dr Williamson wasn't there. The rest I met for the first time.

'You're a little early,' whispered Dr Edwards. 'The lecture hasn't started yet.'

'Damn,' said Dr Oaks.

'Is the lecture before or after dinner?' asked Margaret.

'Before, of course,' said Dr Edwards. 'No one would stay for it if we ate first.'

'Ladies and gentlemen,' called Dr White, banging a spoon on the nearest table and startling a waiter so much that he dropped a trayful of sherry glasses. Fortunately they had all been drained.

The hubbub of conversation slowly died away. We all shuffled noisily into seats.

'Our speaker this evening is the well-known psychiatrist Dr Wainwright,' said Dr White. 'I'm going to be brief because Dr Wainwright needs absolutely no introduction. . . .'

The rest of Dr White's introduction went unheard since the other diners all resumed their previous conversations at these words.

'We had a talk on apathy last time,' said Dr Edwards.

'No one turned up,' complained Dr Oaks.

'Dr Wainwright is the author of numerous celebrated papers,' went on Dr White, 'and a contributor to the *Yearbook of Psychiatric Abstracts.*'

'There was a meeting on schizophrenia before that,' said Dr Edwards.

'I was in two minds about going to that,' said Dr Oaks, 'but in the end I gave it a miss.'

'And so I give you Dr Wainwright,' concluded Dr White. There was a brief round of applause. Dr Wainwright talked for about ten minutes. He told us that he had become a psychiatrist because he couldn't stand smelly feet and that few mental patients take their socks off, and he warned us that if we ever tried to open the cupboard doors behind which our patients store their skeletons we would probably be unable to shake ourselves free of the things for years afterwards.

That is all I remember of his talk. The dinner, however, was more memorable. Dr Oaks said he hadn't eaten such succulent beef for years, and we all had second helpings. The pudding, an imaginative confection of ice cream and fruit, was if anything better.

Dr Edwards, who was looking after my patients as well as his own, was called out only once during the evening. Afterwards Dr Oaks telephoned the local police station and a kindly constable brought his car along.

When we got home both Margaret and I were violently sick, and the next morning we discovered that every doctor who had attended the dinner had contracted staphylococcal food poisoning.

4

WHEN DR OAKS RETIRED his patients were not automatically transferred into my care. They were given the opportunity either to settle under my fledgling wing or to find another more experienced practitioner. Although most chose to stay – acknowledging, I suspect, faith in Dr Oaks' judgement rather than faith in my abilities – some did not. My list shrank noticeably during the first few weeks of the year, and as the postman brought more and more requests from patients asking to be transferred to other doctors I began to fear that the practice would soon disappear altogether.

Two days after the ill-fated clinical dinner, when my stomach hesitantly began once more to acknowledge that eating might soon be possible and even essential again, I decided to call on Dr Oaks, partly to see how he was and partly to ask his advice.

When he'd moved from the surgery Dr Oaks had gone to a small cottage in a nearby village. It was not, as he had threatened, without a telephone or a letterbox, but it was difficult to find and impossible to see from the roadway. Tenacious climbing roses surrounded front door and windows, and rhododendrons filled the tiny garden. Half a dozen sparrows pecked busily at a scatter of breadcrumbs by the door. It seemed that Dr Oaks was well enough to feed the birds.

I hammered on the front door several times before a bedraggled and pyjama'd Dr Oaks poked his head through an upstairs window.

'The door's open,' he croaked miserably. 'Come on in.'

The beams inside were at a head-stunning height, and I walked in with neck bowed. The staircase was directly in front of me, and I climbed up it slowly and with some discomfort. The effects of the food poisoning had left me weak and physically hesitant.

Dr Oaks was sitting in a comfortable easy chair in the bay

window of his bedroom. On a small table stood a half-empty bottle of Perrier water and a glass. An unopened bottle stood on the floor underneath it, and on the arm of the chair a rumpled copy of the *Daily Telegraph* hung precariously.

'I am never, ever eating there again,' he swore with quiet determination.

'I'll not eat there with you,' I promised him.

'How's Margaret?' he asked.

'She's lost five pounds,' I told him. 'And can't make her mind up whether it was worth it or not.'

He managed a slight smile.

'Who's looking after you?' I asked.

'Mrs Law and Miss Jelks have been in with all sorts of potions and damned remedies,' he said. 'Breadcrumbs in water is the latest thing, but I've managed to chuck the stuff out of the window and stick to the Vichy water.' Miss Jelks and Mrs Law, faithful patients who had helped look after Dr Oaks when he lived and worked at the surgery, were clearly not relinquishing their positions of responsibility.

We sat and talked about the iniquities of chefs who serve contaminated food. We briefly discussed the advantages and disadvantages of life in a secluded country cottage, and we mourned the need for modern doctors to hide behind ex-directory telephone numbers, protective receptionists and appointment systems. Eventually I brought up the problem of my disappearing patients.

'How did you build up your practice?' I asked Dr Oaks.

'No magic answer to that, I'm afraid,' he said, pouring himself another glassful of Perrier water. 'It takes time to build up a reputation – although you can lose both within days if you ever step out of line.

'Of course,' he went on, 'when I first went into practice doctors used all sorts of tricks.' He took a large swallow. 'I used to knock on the wrong doors if I had a call to a house in a neighbourhood where I wasn't known too well,' he confessed. 'I'd introduce myself, apologise for the disturbance and go on my way.' He emptied the glass of water and lifted up the un-opened bottle on to his chair-side table. 'That way I picked up quite a few new patients. They remembered my name and called me in when they needed attention.'

I must have looked surprised at his admission.

'I was far less adventurous than most of my colleagues,' he said in self-defence. 'One of them used to ensure that his car broke down at least once a week so that he could pop into the nearest house and ask for help. He'd hang his stethoscope round his neck so they knew immediately that he wasn't the rent collector. And then there was Dr Davidson,' he went on, opening the second bottle and replenishing his glass. 'He used to have his picture in the local paper at least once a week. He was chairman, treasurer or secretary of just about every local organisation. He used to arrange to have himself paged at all the local hotels just to get his name known in the best circles.'

'I thought it was unethical for a doctor to have his picture in a newspaper,' I protested.

'It's perfectly acceptable if he's already well known,' he pointed out. 'And no one ever really knew when Dr Davidson became well known.'

'I can't see myself knocking on the wrong doors, letting the car break down or joining the Women's Institute,' I said sadly. 'I'd be bound to get arrested.'

'You'll pick up patients,' he assured me confidently. 'For the first few months you'll just have to accept everyone who wants you to look after him. In a year or so's time you'll find that your list has increased and you'll be able to refuse the patients who are intent on making your life a misery.'

'Refuse patients?' I said, astonished.

'There are some patients no one wants,' he said. 'They're always in the waiting-room wanting advice, they never do what you tell them and then they blame you if anything goes wrong.'

'How do I know which to reject?' I asked.

'You'll have to decide that for yourself,' said Dr Oaks. 'In fifteen or twenty years' time you'll know instinctively.'

I got back to the surgery to find a message asking me to call on an elderly woman living in two rooms behind the police station. Mrs Hemmings was in her late eighties and as deaf as a milestone. She had several times refused to go into an old people's home where space had been found for her. When I arrived she was sitting in her rocking-chair in front of the television set. The volume control was turned up full, although she was still quite unable to hear anything the commentator was saying. The whole house shook with the starting-prices for the forth-coming race at Newbury.

'Can I turn it down a bit?' I enquired, miming the necessary movement as I spoke.

She looked at me for a moment before nodding slowly. I turned down the volume, leaving the picture alone.

'What's the trouble?' I asked, standing directly in front of her so that she could see my lips.

'Mrs Abberley isn't coming in anymore,' she said.

'Who's Mrs Abberley?' I demanded.

'Mrs Abberley does my shopping for me. She calls in on Mondays, Wednesdays and Fridays and gets my food.'

'Why isn't she coming in anymore?' I asked.

'She's changing her job. She used to work at the cake shop up the way. But she'd had to get a job at the sweet factory.'

I nodded and waited for the rest of the story.

'They have a crush there for the children,' said the old lady.

'A crush?' I asked.

The old lady nodded. Slowly I realised what she meant.

'A crèche,' I corrected her.

'That's what I said,' she shouted. 'A crush.'

'Why has she had to find a crush?' I asked. There are times when it is pointless to argue.

'Her little boy,' she said. 'She has to have someone to look after him.'

'Is his name David?' I asked, suddenly inspired.

'It's David,' she replied. 'David Abberley.'

'The lady who looks after him has had to give it up,' I said.

'There you are,' she said. 'If you know all about it, why are you asking me?'

'Have you got any relatives living locally?' I asked. 'Anyone who could call in and help you?'

She told me that her niece Mrs Liversleigh lived in a village two miles out of town. She gave me the telephone number, and when I got back to the surgery I rang up Mrs Liversleigh to ask if she could help her aunt with shopping and other minor chores.

She was genuinely concerned.

'I'll have her here to live with me,' she offered. 'I've been trying to persuade her to come out here for months.'

'She's very independent,' I said.

'She is indeed,' said Mrs Liversleigh, 'but I'll drive over and talk to her.'

That same evening she rang back to tell me that she had managed to persuade her aunt to leave her small flatlet and live, temporarily at least, with her and her family.

'The only problem is Mrs Hendricks,' she said.

'Mrs Hendricks,' said I. 'Who is Mrs Hendricks?'

'Mrs Hendricks,' she explained, 'is the lady who lives in the flat below my aunt. She's blind and she used to rely on Aunty to help her get along. I don't think she'll be able to manage by herself.'

'You don't happen to know whose patient she is?' I asked.

'She's yours,' replied Mrs Liversleigh instantly.

'I'll go and see her,' I promised.

Mrs Hendricks was in her mid-seventies and almost totally blind. She had developed diabetes in her fifties and, although that problem had been fairly well controlled, she had gone blind in her late sixties. She was a rather bad-tempered old lady who, I later heard, had once hit a newspaper-boy over the head with her white stick for whistling while he worked.

'Have you got any relatives?' I asked her, beginning to wonder where the whole saga was going to end.

'Oh yes,' she said with a noticeable sniff. 'My daughter has an important position.'

'Splendid,' said I.

'She's got a very important job.'

'Marvellous,' I enthused.

'She and her husband live in Northcott Way,' she told me haughtily. 'I think I'll go and live with them.'

'Will that be all right?' I asked.

'Oh yes,' she snapped. 'I'm sure it will. Ring this number.' She handed me a slip of paper. I dialled the number.

'Mrs Knott speaking,' said the woman who answered the telephone.

'This is Dr Vernon,' I said. 'I'm with your mother at the moment.'

'Is she ill?' demanded Mrs Knott.

'She's quite well,' I assured her, 'but there is a bit of a problem. Your mother's friend has moved out this afternoon and your mother has no one here to look after her.'

'Oh dear,' she sighed. 'How boring.'

I felt sure that Mrs Knott's name should mean something, but I'd spoken to so many people and heard so many names that I couldn't remember why.

'I don't like to leave her here by herself,' I said. 'Perhaps you could take her home with you for a few days while we try to sort things out.'

'It's very difficult,' she argued. 'Both my husband and I are out all day. We both have important jobs.'

'It's the night time that's the real problem,' I pointed out. 'Now that Mrs Hemmings has moved out there isn't anyone else in the building.'

'Well, why has Mrs Hemmings moved out?' she demanded.

'It's rather a long story,' I explained. 'Mrs Hollins used to look after David but was told she wasn't certified, so David's mother, Mrs Abberley, had to get another job where she could leave David in a crèche. This meant that she wouldn't be going past Mrs Hemmings' house and therefore couldn't do her shopping. Mrs Liversleigh, who is Mrs Hemmings' niece, has taken her aunt to live with her and that leaves your mother, Mrs Hendricks, on her own.'

'Oh,' said Mrs Knott. 'Is that Mrs Hollins of Wilberforce Street?'

It was then that I remembered where I'd heard of Mrs Knott.

'That's right,' I answered.

'Oh.'

'You see the problem?'

'Quite,' said Mrs Knott.

'What's happening?' demanded Mrs Hendricks crossly. To be honest I'd quite forgotten that she was standing there.

'I'm just explaining things to your daughter,' I told her.

'Is she coming for me?' asked Mrs Hendricks.

'Well, we don't have much option, do we?' said Mrs Knott rather sourly.

'Yes,' I told Mrs Hendricks.

'I should think so too,' said the old lady.

I said nothing. I heard a few days later that Mrs Hollins had suddenly become the proud possessor of a certificate enabling her to look after David Abberley.

Slowly, as the first weeks of my tenure passed, one or two new patients did join the practice. I was flattered by the fact that they had chosen me to look after their health for myself, rather than accepting me simply as successor to Dr Oaks. I did not stop to think that few of them would have left their previous doctor (unless they'd moved home) without there being some discontent, which could as well have been inspired by an unreasonable attitude on the part of the patient as by one on the part of the doctor. Consequently I welcomed Mr Neville to my fold with a warm handshake.

Mr Neville, I discovered later, was in his late thirties, and employed as a medical correspondent by a magazine of national repute. He lived in a small modern detached house on an estate largely housing young executives.

'Good morning, Doctor,' he nodded, when we first met at the end of a morning surgery. He resisted without much apparent difficulty any temptation he might have felt to accompany the greeting with a smile.

I returned the salutation and waited for him to continue.

'Do you have an appointment system?' he asked.

'No,' I told him. 'Not at the moment.'

'You should consider the advantages of providing your patients with an appointment system,' he said.

'I've only just taken over the practice,' I told him. 'I don't want to make any changes at all until I'm rather more established and until I have more of an idea about the advantages which they might bring.' I felt quite proud of that.

'Do you encourage women to have babies at home?' he asked.

'I don't really know,' I had to admit.

'There is a good deal of sound evidence to suggest that home confinements are just as safe as hospital confinements and may be psychologically preferable,' he went on.

'I've not had all that much experience of obstetrics,' I admitted.

'What about prescribing?' he asked. 'What influences do you accept when considering the possible advantages of a new product?'

'Did you want me to treat you for anything?' I asked him, attempting to extricate myself from what was becoming more and more like an in-depth interview.

'Yes, I think so,' he said. 'We'll give you a trial period.'

'Thank you very much,' I replied, in some confusion.

'I have a number of problems which require treatment,' said my new patient, taking a sheet of paper out of his inside pocket.

I said nothing, but folded my arms and waited for him to go on.

'Firstly,' he began, 'I have noticed that between 6.30 a.m. and 12.30 a.m. my urine outflow averages sixty-two ounces.'

'Aha,' said I, having no idea at all of the significance of this statement. I did not even have any real idea how much sixty-two ounces of urine would amount to. It sounded quite a commendable flow.

'Secondly,' went on Mr Neville, 'I have noted that I occasionally have a pain in my wrist during the early hours of the morning.'

'Does it wake you up?' I asked.

'No,' he said firmly.

'Does it keep you awake?'

'No.'

'How long does it last?'

'About two or three seconds.'

'And how many times have you had the pain?' I asked him.

'Twice in all,' he said. 'Once last week and again last night.'

'I don't think that is anything to worry about,' I told him.

'I've also noticed that I have developed a little dandruff,' he continued. This symptom surprised me somewhat since I had already noticed that he wore a toupee. It was not difficult, in fact, to note its existence, since it was three or four shades darker than his remaining hair.

'Whereabouts do you get the dandruff?' I asked him.

'In my eyes,' he said without hesitation. 'There isn't a lot but it's disturbing.'

'I see.'

31

'That's all for now,' he said.

'Right.' I nodded. 'Then I'll prescribe some shampoo for your eyebrows.'

'But I do want to ask you about my children,' he added. 'My son has two small spots on his abdomen. They've been there for twenty-four hours and show no signs of fading.'

'Ah.'

'What do you think it is?' he asked.

'I really don't know,' I confessed.

'Could it be chickenpox?'

'I suppose it could be.'

'My other son has dry skin,' he continued. 'Could you prescribe some cream for him?'

'Certainly.' I was ready to agree to just about anything.

'Finally,' he said, studying his slip of paper carefully, 'my wife has some of the symptoms of a cold.'

'My word,' I remarked.

'I'll hurry up with the symptoms, Doctor,' he said. 'I don't want to bore you.'

He proceeded to describe them in minute detail.

After I'd prescribed a bottle of cough medicine he stood up and removed his coat.

'I wonder if you'd give me a check-up, Doctor,' he said. 'Just for my peace of mind.'

Before I could protest he had stripped to the waist. I decided to listen to his chest and take his blood-pressure before ending the consultation.

'Breathe deeply,' I told him, picking up my stethoscope.

'In or out?' he enquired.

'Yes,' I replied, unable to think of any other answer.

I listened to his chest for a moment or two, heard nothing out of the ordinary and announced my satisfaction. I then unfurled the sphygmomanometer cuff.

'Which arm?' he asked, holding out both hands.

'The left,' I said.

'Oh yes,' he said, nodding in understanding. 'That's the one nearest to the heart.'

'No,' I said, 'it's the one nearest to the sphygmomanometer.'

He said nothing but looked distinctly displeased by my

levity. The rest of the brief examination was completed in silence.

When his medical records arrived from his previous doctor ten days later, I noticed that written in pencil underneath the last entry was the short message, 'Good luck, colleague, whoever you are.'

5

'I'VE HAD MY HUSBAND IN BED for three days and I'm just not satisfied with him,' said Mrs Swann firmly. She sat in the chair on the other side of my desk with her handbag clenched on her lap. She wore a sturdy tweed skirt, a dark-red jumper smeared with chalk marks, and a single string of artificial pearls. When she spoke she peered over the top of tortoiseshell-framed spectacles. The chalk marks made it easy to tell that she earned her living as a schoolteacher. 'He's been having these headaches,' she went on, 'and I really think something ought to be done about him.'

'Well,' I began, intending to point out that since I had heard nothing about her husband's illness until her arrival in the surgery I could hardly be found guilty of neglect for not having offered treatment. Mrs Swann, however, was clearly determined to begin on the attack.

'He's never been ill before,' she interrupted, 'and I think it's a poor job if the doctors can't get him better straight away.'

'We can't — ' I began again.

'All one gets these days are excuses,' she complained. 'It's the same in shops, on the trains, at the post office. I can't remember the last time I had a smile in the post office. The counter clerks there compete to see who can build up the longest queue, and I'll swear the unions rule that the girls must file their fingernails every quarter of an hour.'

'I really don't — ' I started.

'On the railways the ticket clerks and porters seem to regard passengers as unnecessary intruders likely just to leave footprints in the dust in the carriages,' she went on vehemently.

'Has your husband — ?' I tried to ask.

'We pay our taxes and our rates,' she said with a firm nod of her head, agreeing with herself, 'and, although the piper

34

may no longer be able to call the tune, he does like to hear the music occasionally, you know.'

'I agree,' I added quickly.

'Well, if you agree,' she said, 'what are you going to do about my husband?' She opened her handbag, took out a large white linen handkerchief and blew her nose vigorously. It was a genuine professional clearance rather than a timid female gesture.

'Is he fit to come to the surgery?' I asked.

'There you are, you see,' she said, replacing the handkerchief and snapping the bag shut with a firm click. 'Just as I said. Doctors won't do home visits these days. They don't want to know if someone is too ill to get out of bed.'

'I didn't — '

'It is absolutely no good at all trying to wheedle your way out of the pit you've dug for yourself,' she assured me. 'I'm not interested in your excuses. All I want is a fit husband. The lawn has to be cut this weekend, the hedges need trimming and the kitchen ceiling needs repainting.'

'When — '

'It hasn't been done for years,' complained Mrs Swann, 'and it's an absolute disgrace. I don't see how I can be expected to work in a kitchen like that. I spend my days coping with three dozen assorted unruly monsters and I think the least I can expect is a clean kitchen to come home to.'

'Perhaps — '

'Schoolchildren these days are an absolute disgrace,' she said, throwing back her head defiantly, as if I might attempt to contradict her. 'I don't care what anyone says, I see them for seven hours a day and they are an absolute disgrace. They all need whipping. I don't know what their parents think they're doing letting them come to school with such manners. When I was a girl — '

'The address is Gordon Road, isn't it?' I said quickly, as she took a breath. I had noticed that, like many professional politicians, she breathed not at the end of sentences but in the middle, thereby giving those with whom she spoke little opportunity to turn her monologues into a conversation.

'That's right,' she said, thrown a little off balance.

'I'll come along after surgery,' I told her before she could pick up speed again. To indicate that the consultation had come to an end I stood up, walked round the desk, took her by the arm and escorted her to the door. The gesture could have been interpreted as a gentle old-world courtesy, although in truth it was not.

At the end of the evening surgery I got the car out and drove along to Gordon Road. Mr and Mrs Swann lived in a bungalow called Kosy Kot which was neatly sandwiched between a three-storey old people's home and a pub. The front garden was well populated with plastic gnomes. There was one little fellow standing guard over a pair of sorry-looking rose-bushes which had been pruned to death, another clutching a fishing-rod, the distant end of which dangled pointlessly in a crystal-clear pool, a third holding his hat aloft just outside the front door and a fourth leaning lazily against a concrete sun-dial.

The doorbell made a noise such as one might expect to be made by a discordant gnomic orchestra. There were chimings and ringings and lots of tinklings. Mrs Swann opened the front door and immediately stared down at my feet.

'Wipe your feet, Doctor,' she instructed me. 'We've had a new carpet in the hall and it cost £135. Dreadful price.'

I obediently gave the soles of my shoes a few firm strokes on the doormat on the front step.

'And here, if you would,' she said, pointing to a second mat just inside the front door.

I wiped my feet a second time.

'Follow me, Doctor,' she said, closing the front door and bolting it as well. 'I'll take you in to Mr Swann.'

On the right-hand wall of the passage were hung a collection of prints of Paris, showing the Notre-Dame, the Sacré Cœur, the Arc de Triomphe and the Opéra. Between them were hung small three-dimensional plaster casts. There was a brightly coloured cottage, a hunting scene showing a pair of hounds messily despatching a villainous fox, and a farmer leaning on a stile with a pipe in his hand and a piece of straw in his mouth.

Mr Swann was lying in bed. He looked very miserable. There were no glasses of water or fruit juice and no books, magazines or newspapers in sight. His pyjamas were well pressed and the bedsheets were precisely folded.

'Good evening,' I greeted him. 'I'm sorry to hear you've been ill.'

'He still is, Doctor,' said Mrs Swann.

I sat down on the edge of the bed.

'Would you sit here, Doctor?' said Mrs Swann. She moved a chair from the far side of the room and placed it next to the bed. When I got up and obediently sat in it she smoothed the bedclothes again so that the creases I'd created were banished.

'Tell me when it started,' I told Mr Swann.

'Three days ago,' said Mrs Swann.

'Have you been sick?' I asked him.

'No,' said Mrs Swann, 'but you've felt sick, haven't you, George?'

George nodded obediently.

'Can you see all right?'

'He can see all right but he doesn't want to read,' replied Mrs Swann.

'I shall need', I said to Mrs Swann, 'a bowl containing four pints of water at sixty degrees centigrade, a piece of toilet soap, and a towel of some sort not larger than twenty-four inches square.'

'Certainly,' she said. She scurried across the bedroom, opened a drawer and produced a notepad and pencil. She then wrote down my requirements.

When she'd gone I turned to her husband.

'Have you ever had anything like this before?' I asked him.

George Swann shook his head slowly and carefully.

He answered the rest of my questions sensibly enough and I tested his blood-pressure and listened to his chest. His body seemed in perfect condition and I could find no explanation for the headaches. By the time Mrs Swann returned I had finished my examination.

'Here you are, Doctor,' she said. 'I'm sorry I took so long, but your requirements were rather specific.'

'Oh, I'm a bit of a stickler with regard to science,' I told her. 'I find that it pays to be precise.'

'Of course,' she replied. She seemed to approve.

She put the bowl down on the dressing-table and placed a small towel and new tablet of soap by the side of it.

'What did you want all this for, Doctor?' she asked.

'To wash my hands,' I answered, doing just that. 'I'm most grateful to you.'

She seemed rather disappointed at this.

'I don't think there is anything substantially wrong with your husband,' I told her. I put two large white tablets down on the dressing-table. 'I want him to take these straight away,' I told her.

'Will that cure it?' she asked suspiciously.

'If it doesn't,' I told her, 'you must ring me.'

'I shall,' she said, and I had no doubt that she would.

I left the house with a sigh of relief. I'll swear the lazy gnome winked as I left.

Next morning at half-past ten Mrs Swann rang the surgery again.

'My husband is no better,' she announced triumphantly. 'In fact, I think he's worse.'

'Well, I couldn't find anything at all wrong with him,' I told her.

'Does than mean that there *is* nothing wrong with him?' she asked. 'Can you assure me without doubt that you missed nothing?'

I had to admit that I might be mistaken.

'Well, then, I think we ought to have a second opinion, don't you?'

'If you like,' I agreed. 'I'll arrange for someone else to call round later today.'

When she'd put the telephone down I rang Dr White, the consultant physician at the local hospital. He agreed to meet me at the Swanns' bungalow in the afternoon.

His examination was far more thorough than my own. He used pins, needles, hammers and a test tube filled alternately with hot and cold water to test Mr Swann's neurological system. He elicited reflexes I didn't even know existed in places Mr Swann didn't know he'd got. Throughout the examination Mrs Swann provided us all with encouragement.

Eventually Dr White led me into the bathroom for a short discussion. When consulting in a patient's home doctors usually like to find somewhere private to discuss difficult problems. I have in the past had a long talk with a consultant surgeon while standing in a toilet. The surgeon took the only available seat.

'I can't find anything wrong with this fellow,' Dr White admitted, 'but if he's had the blasted headache for four days now we ought to get to the bottom of it. I'll take him into hospital and do an electroencephalogram.'

Mrs Swann seemed almost impressed when we told her that her husband was to go directly into the local hospital. She was even more impressed when told he was to have an electro-encephalogram. I telephoned for an ambulance and, by the time Dr White had repacked the small suitcase in which he carried his equipment, Mr Swann was ready to leave for the hospital.

I didn't expect to hear any more about him for a while, but that evening I got a telephone call from Dr White.

'Your man Swann,' he said, 'made a miraculous recovery this evening. He'd only been in the hospital three hours when his headache disappeared quite spontaneously.'

'Splendid!' I cried. 'What did you do?'

'Nothing,' said Dr White. 'Absolutely nothing.' He paused. 'And don't speak so loud,' he pleaded. 'I've got a splitting head-ache.'

'That's funny,' I said.

'I'm glad you find it so,' he said rather stiffly.

'No, I mean funny odd, not funny ha ha,' I told him quickly. 'I had a headache yesterday evening and I've got another one now.'

The solution to this medical mystery came to us both at once.

'I'll keep this poor beggar Swann in for a week,' said Dr White. 'Give him a bit of a break.'

Mrs Swann was disgusted when I rang her next morning to tell her that her husband was being kept in hospital.

'Who's going to do the kitchen ceiling?' she demanded.

I put the phone down quietly before I developed another headache.

6

GENERAL PRACTITIONERS IN BRITAIN are self-employed. Their income is made up from many different sources. For each patient that a general practitioner agrees to look after the Government pays a small annual sum. There are other small sums for vaccinating young children against polio, diphtheria and tetanus, and for visiting patients during the darker hours of the night.

Most general practitioners do, however, make a little more money outside the health service. Some like Dr Williamson work as industrial medical officers, providing medical advice for companies too small to hire their own full-time adviser. Many do life insurance examinations for insurance companies who suspect that their clients might prove unprofitable. And, of course, all general practitioners are entitled to look after private patients.

There are in fact few advantages in being a private patient. The only two significant ones are that the privately financed doctor is likely to spend more time examining your wart than he would if its disposal were being paid for by the Government and that the doctor will probably visit you at home if you find the prospect of sitting in the waiting-room at the surgery too daunting.

When he retired Dr Oaks had had a couple of dozen private patients who paid him small but welcome sums to visit them at home and pamper their idiosyncrasies. When I took over the practice most of them left it and became patients of one of the other, better-established doctors in the town. I suppose they felt that a young and inexperienced man would hardly be worth paying.

One patient, however, did remain faithful. Mrs Halcyon Melville, a charming, socially superior lady of immense wealth who lived in a huge mansion surrounded by acres of rolling parkland thick with roaming deer, wrote me a very charming letter on heavily embossed notepaper informing me that she would be retaining my services for a trial period of one year. I appreciated her trust, put her letter away in a file of correspondence which I didn't quite know what else to do with and forgot about her completely.

And then, a month or so after my appointment as successor to Dr Oaks, I received a summons to attend her at my earliest convenience. It arrived with the morning mail, and obediently I set off to visit her after morning surgery.

The driveway to her establishment curved majestically across the estate. Its shining white gravel seemed dazzling in even the weakest light and promised to be positively stunning in bright sunshine. Before the house it circled a huge ornamental lake upon which swam rare geese and swans.

The front of the house itself was decorated with pillars and a pair of stone steps which rose in two grand sweeps to a solid iron door. Above that, a huge stone portal was decorated with trumpet-playing nymphs who had themselves been decorated by aesthetically ignorant pigeons.

I parked my car in the centre of the broad sweep of driveway and tiptoed nervously across the gravel and up the steps. Naked, well-endowed, giant females stood guard at the bottom of the steps and a huge pair of stone lions glowered from the top.

The door was embellished with a brass knocker so big that, if melted down, it could have been turned into a church bell. With genuine difficulty I prised it away from the door and let it fall back. The ensuing crash startled me but attracted little attention inside the house. I waited a few minutes, taking the opportunity to absorb the view across the parkland, and tried again. I lifted up the knocker and was about to let it fall again when to my absolute horror I discovered that it had come loose. The hinge at the top which held it on to the door was clearly unequal to the task. Gingerly I lowered the knocker back into place and rapped on the door with my knuckles. As you can imagine, that brought about as much reaction as if a fly had started doing a tap dance. I was about to give up, go back to the surgery and telephone for advice about how best to get in to see Mrs Melville, when the door unexpectedly swung open.

The man who had opened it looked as surprised to see me as I was to see him. He wore a black pinstripe suit and a shirt with a white flyaway collar.

'Good morning,' he said, greeting me rather as he might have been expected to greet a tramp turning up in a parade of elegant dinner guests.

'Good morning.' I smiled, hoping to break down his reserve with a friendly grin. It didn't work.

'If you're looking for work or selling items for the kitchen, please attend at the back door where the housekeeper will see to you,' murmured the man I took to be a butler.

'No,' I told him, 'I'm not looking for work or selling anything.' I took my stethoscope out of its pocket and waved it at him. 'I'm the doctor,' I announced. 'I've come to see Mrs Melville.'

'I believe the rear entrance would be more suitable, sir,' said the butler. 'If you would walk around the house to the right, you will find yourself at the correct door.'

He came out of the house, and closed the door behind him. I noticed to my surprise that he was carrying a small stainless-steel trowel and a wooden box, the sort that seeds are grown in.

The rear entrance was guarded by a plump good-natured woman in a smart white nylon overall. When I had explained who I was she took me through the kitchens and into the main part of the house. I followed obediently as my guide led me up the stairs. At last, some twenty minutes after I'd first arrived at the front door, I found myself facing Mrs Melville.

'Good morning, Doctor,' said my patient with a little nod. She looked to be somewhere between the ages of twenty-five and fifty. I wouldn't have liked to make a more accurate estimate. She wore a pink lacy négligé and reclined on a bed covered with multicoloured cushions.

'What can I do for you?' I asked her, putting my black bag down on the edge of a green velvet chaise-longue. I opened the bag wide, ready for action.

'Sit down,' she said, pointing to a couple of blue cushions

on the side of her bed. She waved imperiously to the house-keeper, who disappeared without another sound.

'So you're Dr Vernon,' she said. She examined me carefully for a few silent moments. I stared back patiently.

A small black and white kitten emerged from underneath one of the cushions on the bed and climbed up on to her lap. I realised then what the butler had been outside to fetch and why the bedroom had a smell not entirely chic.

'Have you any pains?' I asked, hoping to begin my examination.

'Some,' she said enigmatically.

'How long have you had them?' I enquired politely.

'Ages,' she replied. 'Positively ages.'

'A week?'

'Ages.'

'A month?'

'Oh, I don't know.'

'A year?'

'Probably.'

'Do you get sick at all?'

'My legs ache a lot,' she told me inconsequentially.

'It's a big house,' I said, deciding that since the conversation was taking no particular direction there was little point in attempting to ask meaningful questions.

'My husband died two years ago in a road accident,' she said.

'I'm sorry to hear that,' I murmured.

'I wasn't,' she said. She stroked the kitten and picked it up to tickle it under its chin.

'Oh,' I said. Conversations in which I'm an active partner have an uncanny way of moving off on their own in directions I'd rather they didn't take.

'He was lucky with money but unlucky with number twelve buses,' she said. 'Though in a way I suppose he was lucky in that he was run over in front of a hospital.'

'They didn't save him, though?'

'The best way to find all your lost relatives is to be left a great deal of money in a will that is published in all the news-papers,' she said. 'I never knew that my husband or I had so many relatives.'

'I can imagine,' I said.

'My husband's will was rather an unusual one,' she said. 'He remade it every month while he was alive, and the month he died I happened to be suffering from a bad cold. His will stipulated that I should receive income from his estate and be allowed to live in this house for as long as I should remain in poor health.'

I must have looked puzzled.

'My husband felt aggrieved at the time that he was unable to enjoy his conjugal rights,' she explained. 'It was his idea of revenge. If I stay ill, then I live in comfort and style. If I become fit and well, then I live in penury.'

'But you look quite well now,' I blurted out.

'I assure you, Dr Vernon,' she said, 'that my appearance of good health is entirely deceptive.' She put the kitten down and adjusted one or two cushions.

'I'm sorry to hear that,' I commiserated.

'I have over the years been an avid reader of medical journals and a great student of the vagaries of the human body,' she went on.

I couldn't help thinking that she and one or two of my other patients might make good companions.

'Ask me any question you like and I'll answer it,' she boasted.

'I beg your pardon?'

'Ask me a question on a medical topic,' she repeated.

I thought for a moment. 'Where's your appendix?' I asked. 'Can you show me?'

'No,' she said bluntly.

'Aha,' said I. 'Shall I try another?' I smiled condescendingly at her.

'Perhaps you'd better,' she said. 'My appendix was removed when I was six years old and I'm afraid I have absolutely no idea what they did with it.'

I felt myself blushing.

'Of course you'll not know if I'm ill or not,' she said. 'I've become a habitual liar.'

'Really?' I asked, open-mouthed.

'No, not all the time,' she said with a smile.

'How do I know ...?' I began.

'You don't.'

44

I watched the kitten strut past me and disappear off the end of the bed.

'I shall pay you a retainer of a hundred pounds a year and twenty-five pounds a visit to be my doctor,' she said. 'If you ever find me well, your employment will cease.'

'You're asking me to be dishonest,' I said, standing up rather quickly and feeling extremely pompous as I did so.

'You have to sign a small certificate for my lawyers confirming that I am still enjoying bad health,' she said, ignoring my protest.

I stood still, fidgeting with the buttons of my coat.

'If I lose possession of my husband's estate,' she said, 'the entire amount is to be handed over to the Government.'

My bottom jaw fell again.

'My husband had successfully cheated the Government of half a million pounds the month he made that will,' she explained. 'He felt slightly guilty.'

'What's wrong with you at the moment?' I asked her.

'I have a backache.'

'How do I know you are telling me the truth?'

'Are you calling me a liar?'

'No, of course not,' I replied, 'but you did say. . . .'

'I said I lied sometimes,' she said. 'I didn't say I lied all the time.'

'Shall I examine you?' I asked.

'If you must.' She threw a few cushions off the bed and lay down on her back.

'Where is the pain?' I asked her.

'Here,' she said, pointing to the lower part of her back.

'Any pains in your legs?'

She nodded. 'Down the back of my right leg,' she said.

I lifted her leg and tried to move it upwards. She cried out in pain as I lifted it about ten inches off the bed.

'I'm sorry,' I apologised. 'Perhaps we ought to have an X-ray,' I suggested.

'What do you think it is?' she asked.

'A prolapsed intervertebral disc,' I answered. 'Probably.' I paused for a moment. 'Possibly.'

'An X-ray won't prove anything,' she said, 'will it?'

With some reluctance I shook my head. She handed me a

ready-printed certificate which indicated that she was feeling ill. I signed it, snapped my bag shut and waved her goodbye. Fortunately for my future with her I was less than halfway down the stairs when I heard the kitten mewing inside my drug bag. I released it and hurried away.

7

'I HAVE A CALL FOR YOU,' said a lady with a plum-in-the-mouth voice when I picked up the telephone one day in early March. Since the telephone had managed to ring without ceasing while I had ignored it, climbed out of the bath, wrapped a bath-towel around myself and dripped my way into the bedroom, her statement seemed a likely possibility.

'If you'll just hang on,' said the voice, 'Major Whitbee will be with you in just one minute.'

I am continually amazed by the way in which the telephone has affected our lives. If one user wishes to speak to another, surely it is impertinent for him to arrange for a secretary or aide to see that he picks up the telephone receiver only when the conversation is ready to begin. I can understand busy people's using operators and secretaries for time-consuming long-distance calls necessitating tiring digital exercises, but I never fail to be angered by people who keep me waiting when the call is local and unlikely to involve any great delay. I become particularly upset when I am interrupted in mid-meal or mid-bath and kept waiting while the caller completes apparently more urgent business. If I had been alive when Alexander Graham Bell was busy inventing the telephone, I think I would have urged him to invent something else. Any murderous weapon would have my blessing in place of an instrument which has in its time surely destroyed more good meals and wasted more gallons of warm water than any other piece of technological wizardry.

'Hullo, Major Whitbee's secretary,' whispered a second plum-in-the-mouth voice.

'Hullo?' I called back, pulling the towel a little tighter.

'Who is that, please?'

I gave my name.

'Whom did you want?' demanded Major Whitbee's secretary, clearly something of a pedant.

'You rang me.' The bedroom carpet was beginning to change colour and my goose pimples were acquiring goose pimples of their own.

Eventually the lady who had described herself as Major Whitbee's secretary discovered that she had indeed initiated the call and with tremendous generosity she agreed to put me through to the mysterious man himself.

'Major Whitbee will speak to you in just a moment,' she told me breathlessly.

'Excuse my curiosity,' I begged, 'but could you please tell me who Major Whitbee is?'

'I beg your pardon?' asked the great man's secretary.

'I have never heard of your Major Whitbee,' I told her. 'Should I have?'

'Major Whitbee,' said the plum-voiced lady in awe, 'is the hospital secretary.'

'Which hospital is that?' I asked, in honest innocence.

'The John Taylor Hospital for the Mentally Disabled,' she replied. She sounded as dismayed as if I'd denied knowledge of the existence of the Queen or John Wayne.

'Here is Major Whitbee,' she said at last, still aghast at my ignorance.

'Good day to you, Doctor,' boomed a cheery masculine voice.

'To whom did you wish to speak?' I enquired as politely as I could.

'Dr Vernon,' answered the Major, rather surprised.

'Speaking,' I told him. 'What can I do for you?'

'I believe you took over Dr Oaks' practice earlier this year?' he began.

'That's right,' I agreed, shivering.

'Dr Oaks was on our committee for many years,' he said. 'Now that he's retired he's written to us to tell us that he'll be unable to serve with us in the future.'

I grunted without commitment.

'Of course we shall miss him,' said Major Whitbee. 'He's been a great friend of the hospital.'

'Of course,' I murmured politely.

'It was Dr Oaks himself who suggested that I should ring you and invite you to take his place,' he told me.

'On the committee?' I asked.

'Exactly.'

'What committee is that?' I asked, silently cursing Dr Oaks.

'The Hospital Management Committee,' he answered. 'It meets once every two months.'

'Well, I'm very flattered . . .,' I started, about to ask for time to consider his suggestion.

'Good, well, that's settled, then,' he said without delay. 'We'll be sending you details of the hospital, of course, but perhaps you'd be able to come along to our next meeting.'

'I'll certainly try,' I told him. 'It's difficult, you understand, with my practice commitments.'

'That's no problem,' he said. 'The hospital is only about five miles from your surgery. Your staff can reach you here by telephone at any time.'

'Thank you,' I told him meekly.

'The next meeting is this afternoon,' he told me.

'This afternoon?'

'At half-past three. We'll look forward to seeing you.'

I put down the telephone and walked back into the bathroom.

'Who was that?' asked Margaret when I went downstairs. 'Your breakfast has been ready for ages.'

I told her.

'Congratulations,' she said. 'I've put the milk on your cornflakes, so you'd better hurry up or else they'll be horribly soggy.'

At fifteen minutes past three I abandoned the huge pile of correspondence which I'd been ploughing through. Before I'd inherited the practice I had seen comparatively little of the avalanche of paper under which general practitioners are frequently buried and lost. While I had been working as his assistant, Dr Oaks had still dealt with the mail, answering communications from insurance companies, replying to letters from health service administrators and reading miscellaneous correspondence from hospitals and relatives. When I'd assumed full responsibility for the practice I had also taken over the

49

mail. It was a chore I could easily have managed without. My first reaction was to attempt to deal with everything as it arrived; my later reaction was to leave all non-clinical mail for one month. By that time much of it could be discarded as out of date.

As I was about to leave the house Margaret called to me.

'The fridge door has broken,' she cried rather desperately. 'It won't shut properly.'

'What happened to it?' I asked, halfway through the front door.

'I don't know,' she said sadly, 'but it just won't shut, and all the food will go rotten.' She was almost in tears.

'Give Mr Enstone a ring,' I told her. 'He's an electrician with a hernia.'

With that I kissed her and abandoned her.

The hospital was a typical large Midland mental hospital. A huge village of a place, built in several acres of parkland a mile or two out of town, it was an architectural potpourri of nineteenth-century red-brick buildings and twentieth-century prefabricated bungalows. It's a sign of the progress we've made in the last century that the older buildings are sturdy and weatherproof and the newer buildings shake in the wind and leak when it rains.

As I drove up the winding drive which wriggled its way between a series of huge oak-trees I noticed a man running towards me. I slowed down to avoid a collision and watched him run past me and begin to clamber up a nearby tree.

When I reached the end of the drive I parked in a small square which was almost filled with expensive-looking vehicles. I was locking the car when two men in white coats burst through the front doors of the main building and dashed out into the car-park.

'Have you seen a man come rushing out of here?' demanded one as I wandered over towards them.

I nodded.

'Where did he go?' asked the second.

'Down the drive,' I told them.

They both started off.

'He climbed one of the trees,' I called after them.

They stopped suddenly and came back towards me.

'Which tree?' they asked together.

Now, it's a funny thing, but trees, like Chinamen, look very much the same at first glance. It's difficult to tell one oak-tree from another oak-tree. I walked back down the drive but couldn't for the life of me find the right tree.

Just as we were about to abandon the search a shoe landed six feet away from one of the two white-coated men. Instinctively we all looked up and were just able to move away as a second shoe landed between us.

'There he is!' called one of the men, pointing up at the topmost branches. The fugitive waved cheerily.

'Who is he?' I asked.

'That's George,' explained the man, as if that were sufficient. 'He's one of our patients. He decided he didn't want to have his hair cut today. He's always running off.'

'I'll stay here with him, Bert,' said the other man. 'You go back and fetch a ladder.'

I walked back up the drive with Bert. At the front door we met a tall thin man growing through his hair. He wore a neat moustache, a pair of gold-rimmed spectacles and a loud-checked three-piece suit.

'What's going on?' he demanded frostily.

'George has climbed a tree, Major,' said Bert timidly.

'Well, get a ladder and get him down,' ordered the Major. 'We have a committee meeting this afternoon.' He looked at me. 'Visiting-time isn't until seven today,' he said firmly.

'I've come — ' I began.

'I'm sorry about that,' said the Major. 'Get that ladder straight away, Busby,' he snapped at the man standing beside me. I watched him fetch a ladder and carry it back down the drive. The operation seemed to promise more than the committee meeting in the way of entertainment.

Unfortunately for us all, the ladder reached only about half-way up the tree. Although both white-coated men climbed up, they found they could get nowhere near to George, who was safely ensconced in a fork at the top. And George could have got nowhere near to the ladder even if he had wanted to.

The two men came back up the drive together this time. The

Major was still standing at the door greeting committee members as they arrived.

'The ladder won't reach,' said Busby.

'We need the fire brigade,' said the other.

'Well, call them!' ordered Major Whitbee. 'And get on with it.' He seemed upset.

I hung back, anxious to see the remainder of the episode and not too keen to sit at a table with Major Whitbee.

'What's going on down there?' demanded the Major suddenly. He pointed down the drive to where a group of twenty or thirty patients, some of them dressed in pyjamas, had gathered at the foot of one of the oak-trees. As we watched one of them began to clamber up the ladder.

By the time the two white-coated men had got back down the drive all the patients had disappeared. We discovered, as a shower of shoes and slippers rained about us, that they were all sitting in the uppermost branches of neighbouring oak-trees.

The arrival of the fire brigade was spectacular. Whoever had called for help had clearly not given specific information and the six fire-engines were accompanied by three ambulances and two police cars.

'Where is it?' demanded a fireman, leaping from the leading engine.

'They're up there,' said Bert, pointing upwards.

The fireman seemed puzzled.

'Some patients of ours are up a tree,' he explained.

'Up several trees,' explained his colleague.

In the distance I saw Major Whitbee, red-faced with fury, trying to shepherd his committee members indoors. They seemed reluctant to leave.

One of the fire-engines drove directly underneath the tree up which George had climbed. A fireman clambered up his ladder and tried to persuade him to come down. George, enjoying his new-found status, was not interested.

It was at this stage that I decided to go back home. I climbed into my car and threaded my way back down the drive between the fire-engines, ambulances and police cars. By this time an army of experts were scratching their heads.

When I got back to the surgery Margaret rushed to greet me.

'I'm sorry,' she said. 'I'm so stupid.'

I looked at her in puzzlement.

'Mr Enstone said he wouldn't charge us,' said Margaret. 'He was very understanding.'

'Mr Enstone?'

'The electrician,' explained Margaret. 'He came to mend the fridge door.'

'Oh yes,' I agreed. 'Did he manage it?'

Margaret nodded, blushing.

'What was wrong with it?' I asked her.

'I bought some cucumbers this morning,' said Margaret. 'And one of them was too long to fit inside.'

'That's why the door wouldn't shut?' I asked her.

She nodded. 'I cut it in two,' she told me. 'It's all right now.'

8

SOME PATIENTS are belligerent and angry because they are frightened and worried. Others are belligerent and angry because they are rude, aggressive people. Councillor Hugh Wells fell into the latter category.

In principle he worked as a machine-tool operator at the local cardboard box factory, but in practice most of his time was spent on political and semi-political activities. He was the local representative of the Cardboard Box and Paper Bag Workers' Amalgamated Union, and a leading light in the local Labour Party, as well as a councillor and chairman of the Housing Committee.

I first met him one Wednesday in March when he came to see me complaining of a bad back.

'I've come with my legs, Doctor,' he said. He waved one leg in the air while he leant on the wash-basin. 'I can't use this one at all for the pain.'

I asked him some straightforward questions about the pain and discovered that he had been troubled with backache for nearly three weeks.

'It's just getting worse and worse,' he complained. 'I can hardly swing a golf club.'

'What do you think caused it?' I asked him innocently.

'I'm glad you asked me that, Doctor,' he said, wagging a finger at me. 'I'm a victim of capitalist exploitation.'

I asked him what he meant.

'I did my back in at the factory,' he said.

'What happened?' I asked.

'I was carrying a pile of work about,' he complained, 'and the foreman wouldn't give me anyone to help.'

'What sort of work?' I asked, making notes.

'Paper,' he explained. 'I was moving union records into my new office.'

I suggested that a week's rest and some pain-killing tablets might prove beneficial.

He was not impressed.

'Don't you think I ought to see a specialist?' he asked.

'I don't think so,' I told him. 'Not at this stage.'

'Would you give me a letter to our solicitor?' he enquired.

'Solicitor?' said I.

'I shall be taking action against the company,' he informed me.

'I don't know that there's anything much I can write to help you,' I told him.

'Just a note to the effect that I have a bad back,' he said. 'That'll do.'

I picked up a piece of notepaper and began to write a short referral letter.

'You might just add that I got the bad back at work,' he said.

I obediently completed the letter.

'Do you think you'll really have much of a case?' I asked him.

'My cousin is in the House of Commons,' he said.

'Is he?' I said, impressed.

'He's been in the Commons for years,' added the Councillor.

'What's his name?' I asked, thinking that perhaps I might have heard of him.

'Michael O'Flanery,' replied Councillor Wells.

I shook my head. 'I don't think I've heard of him,' I admitted.

'You'll not have done,' he agreed. 'He's a bit of a backroom boy.'

'A backroom boy?' I asked.

'He doesn't get into the limelight much.'

'What exactly does he do?' I asked, curious by now.

'Well, he's a communications expert,' said the Councillor.

'Communications,' I said. 'Very important.'

'He helps transmit vital messages around the Commons,' Councillor Wells confided.

'Really?' I said.

'He's called a messenger,' said Councillor Wells, 'but it's a very responsible job.'

'I'm sure it is,' I agreed. I put the letter into an envelope and handed it to him after sealing it.

'Thank you,' he said, taking his letter, his sick-note and his prescription.

The next patient was the local vicar, the Reverend Dewhurst.

'My problem is a rather embarrassing one,' he said with a nervous cough.

I nodded, encouraging him to continue.

'It's hardly a medical problem,' he insisted with diffidence.

'Go on,' I told him.

'I think perhaps I ought to leave it.'

'It's up to you,' I told him.

'I'll leave it,' he said, standing and preparing to go.

'Wouldn't it be better to get it off your chest?' I asked him.

'It's my arm, not my chest,' he said.

Puzzled, I looked at him.

'I suppose you might be able to help,' he murmured, hoping for more encouragement.

'I will if I can,' I promised.

He sat down again. Just then there was a gentle knock on the door. It was Miss Williams.

'I've brought you some tea and biscuits,' she said, with an unexpected smile in the vicar's direction.

'Oh, thank you,' I managed to say. Miss Williams was not in the habit of bringing tea or biscuits into the surgery while patients were present.

The vicar waited until she had gone and then moved his chair a little closer to the desk.

I waited expectantly.

'Shall I pour?' he asked, pointing to the tea-pot.

'Please do,' I told him.

We both sipped our cups of tea.

'May I take a biscuit?' he asked.

'Please do,' I repeated.

'It's very nice tea,' he noted.

'Yes.' I smiled.

'I was in the Army during the war,' he told me unexpectedly.

'Ah.'

'In Turkey.'

I made some sound of mild encouragement.

'And Malta,' he went on. 'It happened in Malta.'

'Ah.'

'Some of the fellows in my battalion found out that it was my birthday and insisted on having a little party in my honour.'

'A birthday party.' I smiled.

'That's right,' he said. 'I don't have birthday parties now but I sometimes think it's rather a pity.' He reached for another biscuit. 'I think I'd rather like playing some of the games we played when we were children,' he explained. 'Blind man's buff, hide and seek, and so on.'

There was a silence for a few moments while we both finished our biscuits.

'More tea, Vicar?' I asked, lifting the pot and offering to pour.

'I will, thank you,' he said. He stared for a moment as I filled his cup. 'You know, I didn't use to like tea,' he told me, 'but I must have drunk thousands of gallons of it in the last twenty years. I remember a bishop of mine once telling me that, if clergymen stopped drinking tea, he felt sure that our balance of payments would remain permanently in the black.'

'It happened in Malta,' I reminded him.

'Did it?' he asked. 'What was that?' He looked up at me. 'I was in Malta, you know.'

'You were going to tell me something that happened there.'

'Oh yes,' he said. 'At my birthday party.'

I nodded and waited.

'I got tattooed,' he said suddenly.

'Ah,' I said, understanding at last.

'Some of the fellows got me a little tiddly and took me along to a tattooing parlour. I woke up next morning and had the fright of my life.'

'What was it?' I asked.

'A tattoo,' he explained.

'I mean, what was the tattoo?' I asked.

'Well, it was a lady,' he stammered. 'A lady unveiled as you might say.'

'A nude,' I suggested.

'That's it,' he said. 'I *am* glad I told you.' He breathed a huge sigh of relief and rolled up his left sleeve. On his forearm there was a large blue tattoo of a naked lady with a pair of breasts sticking out at an angle which would have defied gravity, Brunel and Howard Hughes.

57

'There you are,' he said. 'Can you help me?'

'What do you want me to do?'

'I want it rubbed out.'

'It's not that easy,' I said. 'I think you can probably have it removed, but you'll have to see a plastic surgeon and have skin grafting.'

'They can do it, though?'

'Yes, I think so.'

'That's marvellous,' he said. 'I'll put our balance of payments in further peril and have another cup of tea.'

We were halfway through our third when there was a second knock on the surgery door. This time it was Margaret.

'Oh, I'm sorry,' she said. 'I didn't know you had anyone with you.'

'That's perfectly all right,' said the vicar, hastily rolling down his sleeve. 'I was just going.'

'It's those pictures I bought,' said Margaret. 'I wondered if you'd hang them for me.'

'Oh dear,' I moaned politely. 'I'll try, but I doubt if I'll be able to get them straight.'

When Dr Oaks had left he hadn't taken all the furniture but he had removed all the pictures, and the blank walls looked terrible.

'Aha,' said the vicar, his forefingers held aloft. 'Then you must allow me to help. Hanging pictures is a little skill of mine.' He smiled secretively.

'I'll go and get them,' said Margaret without hesitation, and she disappeared.

'You'll not tell anyone about this, will you?' whispered the vicar, tapping his forearm. 'No one else knows.'

'Of course not,' I told him. 'I'll write the letter of referral in longhand myself,' I promised, 'and you can pick it up and deliver it to the hospital.'

'Perhaps you could make it a hospital some way away?' he suggested.

'I'll do that,' I promised. 'There isn't a plastic surgeon at the local hospital anyway.'

The picture-hanging proved easier than I had feared. To an experienced handyman this is undoubtedly a task that would be classified as 'routine'. To a novice who has to try hard to remember which way to turn a screwdriver when tightening, it is fraught with dangers. It isn't just the possibility of smashing the glass, making holes in the wall or destroying the plumbing that worries me. It is the very real danger that when I've finished the pictures will look as though they were hung by a drunken man with a limp during a gale.

The vicar had the answer. He promised to see to it that even on the stairs our pictures were hung in a perfectly straight line.

'You simply use your nose,' he explained, taking the hammer and nail from me.

I looked at him in horror. I have a fondness for my nose, inspired by years of close contact.

'Stand against the wall,' he told me, 'with your toes touching the skirting-board, and your eyes staring straight ahead.' He did so as he spoke. 'Now move forward until your nose touches the wall,' he said. 'Then put your nail into the wall at the precise spot where the tip of your nose is resting. And make sure you move your nose first.'

He hammered in the first nail.

'Now you try it,' he suggested.

Between us we hung the twenty-four pictures that Margaret had bought and then fetched her to look at the result.

'Very good,' she said without much enthusiasm.

'You're not very happy about it,' I said. 'What's the matter?'

'Why did you hang them in that wavy line?' she asked.

I stood back and looked at the pictures. She was right. They were hanging in a very wavy line. It was regularly wavy, but wavy nevertheless.

'What went wrong?' I asked the vicar.

He frowned and scratched his ear.

It came to us both at once.

'Your pictures are in a straight line,' I said.

'And so are yours,' said the vicar.

We took out the nails he'd hammered in and then I put them back into the wall in line with my nose.

When the Reverend Dewhurst had gone I went back into the surgery to deal with some of the accumulated mail which had begun to smother my desk. As I sorted through half a hundred missives from the moguls of the pharmaceutical industry Miss Williams appeared to clear away the tea things.

'A wonderful man, the vicar,' she said.

'Indeed.'

'Not ill, I hope?'

'No.'

'Having his tattoo off, is he?'

I looked at her open-mouthed.

'He thinks no one knows about it,' she whispered confidentially.

It was just after midnight when I heard from Councillor Wells again.

'My back's giving me a lot of trouble,' he complained on the telephone.

'Have you taken your pills?'

'I'm afraid I haven't,' he confessed. 'I've been rather busy today with a Housing Committee meeting. I didn't manage to get to a chemist's shop.'

'I see,' I replied sleepily.

'I wondered if you could bring me some round,' he suggested.

'Can you not wait until the chemist's open again?' I asked.

'Oh no,' he said, quite flatly. 'Oh no.'

I noted down his address. Reluctantly, but knowing that if I didn't go I'd be called later in the night and form the subject of a report to the union's solicitors, I drove off to his home.

He was busy when I arrived.

'Come in, Doctor,' he called, as his wife let me into the house. 'I'll be with you in just a moment.' His wife showed me into the living-room where he was poring over a huge sheaf of papers.

'It's been dreadful this evening,' he said.

'Have you got the prescription I gave you?' I asked.

He searched on the desk for a moment or two and eventually unearthed it. He handed it to me.

'What's happened to you?' I asked him, nodding towards the back of his right hand which looked badly burnt.

'Oh, nothing much,' he said dismissively. I thought the gesture slightly out of character.

'Let me have a look.'

Reluctantly he held out the hand for me to examine.

'How on earth did you do this?' I asked him.

'Oh, I'm not sure now.'

'You must have done it today.'

'Yes,' he agreed.

'You must know how you did it,' I insisted.

'I got it caught in the steam from the kettle,' he admitted.

'Very nasty,' I said. 'It ought to be dressed.'

'Oh, well, thank you very much, Doctor,' he said.

I didn't tell him that as he'd rummaged through the papers on his desk I'd caught sight of the letter I'd written that morning. The envelope had been steamed open.

'I'll have to take you back to the surgery,' I told him. 'I haven't got anything with me to dress that.'

We both climbed into the car. It was just beginning to rain a little as we left. At the surgery I wrapped a clean bandage around his hand and gave him a small bottle of pain-killing tablets for his back.

'That's very good of you, Doctor,' he said.

'Not at all,' I insisted, ushering him towards the front door.

'Much appreciated,' he added.

I let him out. He waited on the doorstep for a moment.

'Good night,' I cried cheerily, shutting the door and leaving him with a three-mile walk home. I heard some unhappy mutterings from him before I went back to bed.

9

AT LAST the cricket season arrived. All over the country cricketers were lovingly oiling their bats, cleaning their pads and boots, and picking the mothballs out of their chunky white sweaters. Wives and girl-friends were equally active flexing sandwich-spreading fingers and hunting around in the kitchen cupboards for the vacuum flask.

'I've got tickets for the match on Saturday,' said Dr Oaks unexpectedly one Monday evening. 'Want to come?'

I told him I'd have to try to fix up someone to look after the practice and immediately rang Dr Edwards. Fortunately he was planning to visit the London Boat Show, and I was able to arrange a swap. He'd look after my patients while I went to the match, and I'd have his flock under my wing while he peered into boats he couldn't afford even to dream about. I rang Dr Oaks back and told him the good news.

'Pick you up at nine,' he promised.

By the time Friday evening had arrived I was ready for a day away. It had been a hard week. On Tuesday morning there had been a telephone call at five to nine from a Mr and Mrs Unstance who wanted me to go and see their six-month-old baby. They said it was urgent and couldn't possibly wait until surgery was over.

The baby had a cold and needed no treatment at all. By the time I got back to the surgery there were thirty people waiting and murmuring unhappily. I'd seen half of them when Mrs Unstance rang again. She said the baby was still coughing. I pointed out that it would probably cough for a day or two. She said it was my responsibility. I said I realised that. She said that she and her husband wanted another visit.

I told them I'd visit again after surgery had finished, and Mrs Unstance slammed the receiver down so hard that my head rang for several moments afterwards. My hand moved towards the buzzer, ready to summon the next patient, but my finger never got there. Perhaps, I thought, I had made a mistake. Perhaps the baby was really ill. Perhaps it needed urgent help. I knew I wouldn't be able to live with myself if the General Medical Council and the Sunday newspapers let me try. I got back into the car and drove off to the Unstance baby.

It was, of course, fast asleep when I arrived, and was as well as any baby I have ever seen. I muttered encouragement and hurried back to the surgery.

They didn't ring again until three in the afternoon. I was struggling through a huge pile of mail at the time, trying to catch up with directives from the Department of Health, further exhortations from the drug companies and the more important messages from the hospital consultants.

'You'll have to come again,' said Mr Unstance. 'The baby's coughing.'

'The baby's bound to cough a little,' I said. 'He has a cold.'

'It isn't right,' said Mr Unstance. He began again to describe in uncomfortable detail the future that awaited me should I have made the slightest error. Although this time I was quite convinced that there was nothing for me or the Unstances to worry about, I knew that sometimes babies deteriorate rapidly. I got into the car again.

The baby was sitting up taking its feed when I arrived.

'We're not happy about him,' said Mrs Unstance. 'We think he ought to be in hospital.'

'In hospital?' I said, surprised. 'Surely not.'

'We think so,' said Mr Unstance firmly. 'That's what hospitals are for.'

I told them that hospitals are places for the sick and that I didn't think their baby was sick. They seemed determined to ignore my every explanation. I left them both at half-past three and drove back to the surgery exhausted, angry and frustrated.

They rang again at six, just as I was getting towards the end of an unusually light evening surgery.

'The baby isn't any better,' said Mrs Unstance.

'I told you that he won't get better straight away.'

'We want him in hospital. We aren't happy.'

'I really don't — '

'Are you refusing us the right to a second opinion?' she demanded. 'We're entitled to a second opinion, you know.'

'I know,' I agreed.

'So you'll fix him up with a hospital bed,' she said. 'Surely it's up to us to decide when a second opinion is needed.'

I gave up and agreed to arrange for their baby to be admitted to the children's ward at the local hospital.

'Will you send an ambulance?' she asked.

'Can't you take him along?' I asked. 'The ambulances are very busy, you know.'

'That's what ambulances are for, isn't it?' she snapped. 'Petrol costs money, you know. If the baby needs to go into hospital, I don't see why we shouldn't have an ambulance.'

I gave up that battle as well and telephoned for an ambulance. Then I rang the house officer in charge of the children's ward and explained that, although I didn't feel that young Mr Unstance really needed to be in hospital, I just wasn't able to keep him at home any longer. Fortunately the house officer was understanding. He had perhaps had experience himself of people like the Unstances.

Half an hour later Mrs Unstance was on the telephone again.

'The ambulance hasn't arrived yet,' she complained.

'I have rung them,' I told her, 'but they may be coping with a genuine emergency.'

'Ours is an emergency. It's nearly a quarter to seven.'

'Has the baby deteriorated?' I asked.

'Well, no,' she admitted, 'but we've got to be ready for seven. Our friends are picking us up then.'

'Pardon?' I said.

'We've got friends picking us up.'

'You're going out?'

'We're going out to a party.'

'Well, couldn't your baby-sitter stay with the baby until the ambulance arrives?'

'We couldn't get a baby-sitter,' she said.

I put the telephone down as gently as I could.

On Thursday I was in trouble with Mrs Parks. She wanted to have her baby at home and I wanted her to have it in hospital. I explained that it is sometimes all right for women to have babies at home but that, if there is the slightest risk of anything going wrong, then it is safer for both mother and child to be where the equipment and staff are ready to cope with crises.

'What's going to go wrong?' asked Mrs Parks.

I said that I hoped nothing would go wrong, but that her previous baby had been delivered by forceps.

'Mrs Gainsborough had her baby at home and she had a forceps delivery,' said Mrs Parks, trumping my ace very neatly.

'I'm sorry,' I said, quite genuinely, 'but I'm afraid I'm not an obstetrician and I don't feel able to look after you at home should you need anything more than ordinary medical care.'

'Well, if you can't cope with emergencies, what sort of doctor are you?' she demanded.

To that I could think of no answer except to point out that I was not an expert in any field of medicine and that when expert attention was needed I always liked to have specialist advice.

Mrs Parks remained unconvinced and left the surgery announcing that she was off to find another doctor who was qualified to look after her.

On Friday I spent the day looking forward to Saturday, which came round just as slowly as it always does. Next day I jumped out of bed at eight and rushed across the bedroom to fling open the curtains and see what the weather was like. It was raining.

'Never mind,' said Dr Oaks when he arrived. 'It'll probably clear up later on.'

'Shall we go in my car?' I asked, hoping he'd agree so that I wouldn't have to nurse my heart through a couple of hours of sitting beside him at the wheel.

'No, we'll use mine,' insisted Dr Oaks. 'Give you a rest.'

'Thank you,' I murmured meekly.

'Mind how you go,' said Margaret, putting a huge pile of sandwiches in my hands. 'That's just for nibbling.' She gave me a kiss and pecked Dr Oaks on the cheek. 'Do you want a flask of coffee?' she asked, just as we were about to leave.

'I've got one in,' said Dr Oaks. He winked at me but until later, I didn't find out why.

At the ground the crowds were standing around in the bars and huddled together under umbrellas. Play was delayed, so an announcement over the loudspeaker system informed us, until the umpires had inspected the pitch and assessed its suitability for play.

'Drink?' asked Dr Oaks, taking the top off his vacuum flask and handing me a paper cup he'd produced from his coat pocket.

'Thank you.'

He poured me a cupful of steaming hot coffee, which I sipped gratefully. It was bitterly cold, and the coffee seemed to warm me very effectively.

We walked around the ground munching sandwiches. Margaret had supplied us as for a siege. There were fish-paste sandwiches, tuna-fish sandwiches, salad sandwiches, egg sandwiches, cheese sandwiches, beef sandwiches, salmon sandwiches, chicken sandwiches, ham sandwiches, and, incongruously, plum-jam sandwiches. As we walked we talked about the merits of the two teams, we discussed the intellectual disabilities of the county selectors and we rubbed our hands together briskly to get them into shape for clapping should the cricket start. Cricket spectating is a tricky art. The knack is to know precisely when to clap and just how much noise to make. A maiden over, for example, does not merit quite so much applause as a good boundary shot but usually brings slightly more than a partnership of fifty runs put together by two batsmen on an easy pitch.

We walked round the ground twice more. Stopping at the same wall to take a drink of coffee. After the second circuit Dr Oaks peered into the flask with dismay.

'Empty,' he groaned.

'Pity,' I agreed.

'Good job I've got another one in the car,' he said. 'We'll pop over and get it.'

He had parked his car in the club car-park in a spot clearly marked as reserved for the club president. When we got to it a couple of attendants were peering into it while a white-haired man with an unhealthily red face, half-in and half-out of a very expensive-looking Jaguar, shouted at them to move the car out of his way.

'I told you we shouldn't have left it there,' I muttered to Dr Oaks.

'Don't worry,' he said, comfortingly patting me on the hand. He walked boldly over to the two attendants. What he said to them I don't know, but they saluted him when he came back clutching his battered old black bag.

'Put the second flask in here,' he whispered. 'Thought it looked better.' He hurried on and I followed close behind him.

The rain continued to fall lightly. The inspection of the pitch gave us very little hope that there would be any play at all. The highlights of the afternoon were two appeals made over the loudspeaker system. The first brought tremendous cheers from the scattered, slightly damp crowd.

'Would Mr Harris,' said the announcer, 'who has a number of admission tickets for his friends, please go to the main gate where they are waiting for him?'

The second brought even greater cheers.

'Would Mr Wilkins please note that his wife has just given birth to a healthy son. If he could find a spare moment during the day, would he please visit the nursing home?'

Dr Oaks and I celebrated both announcements with a drink of black coffee. I found myself cheering quite wildly at the second.

At four we decided that there would be no play that day. The sky had begun to cloud over and, even if the drizzle did finally stop, it seemed unlikely that the light would be good enough to start a match. It sometimes seems a miracle that cricket matches ever take place at all.

As we got into the car, having emptied the second flask, I felt thoroughly relaxed and rested. The good company, the lack of ringing telephones and the total absence of tiresome folk such as the Unstances had all contributed to an excellent day.

'A friend of mine runs a nursing home near here,' said Dr Oaks as he drove out of the ground. An attendant on the main gate saluted as we left. 'Mind if we call in and say hullo?'

'Not at all,' I said. 'Good idea.'

It must have been near the ground, for I remember very little of the journey. The next thing I recall is stopping outside the Happyrest Nursing Home.

'Woops,' I said as I bumped the door into the immaculate paintwork of a Rolls-Royce.

'Never mind,' said Dr Oaks, who didn't much care what his car looked like as long as it kept him dry and got him from one place to another before it was too late.

'Want you to meet my successor, Dr Vernon,' he said when we'd been shown into a magnificent office by a young nurse in an extremely smart blue uniform.

'Pleased to meet you,' oozed the proprietor.

'This is Nigel,' said Dr Oaks. 'Nigel Baker.'

I took his outstretched hand and winced as he attempted to turn my fingers into mincemeat.

'Would you like to see round?' he asked.

'Love to,' said Dr Oaks.

'Thank you,' I agreed. As we left the office I tripped over a thick Indian carpet. For some reason the incident just made me laugh. I stopped laughing only as we were shown into one of the patient's room.

'These are colleagues of mine,' said Dr Baker, introducing us to an elderly woman in a hideous pink nightdress. We exchanged polite smiles. 'Loaded,' he whispered to me as I sat in a comfortable armchair. For some reason I felt extremely sleepy. 'Examine her, if you like, and we'll put ten guineas on her bill.'

'Is it time for my injection?' asked the lady in pink.

Dr Baker looked at his watch and nodded. He walked across to a cupboard above the sink, unlocked it and removed a small phial.

'Dr Baker has this medicine specially flown in from Germany for me,' said the lady. 'It's wonderful.'

I couldn't help noticing that the phial contained a mystical substance called 'distilled water' and had been manufactured and packaged in Surbiton.

We stayed for another quarter of an hour or so. Dr Baker showed us with understandable pride the expensive X-ray and laboratory equipment that our local hospital would never have been able to afford. Just about the only things missing were patients in genuine need of such significant diagnostic and therapeutic aids. Dr Baker's patients were mostly like the lady in the pink nightdress. There was also an extraordinary man who had changed his name to Mr X and made a fortune from suing newspapers and other wealthy organisations for libelling him. He had finally suffered an acute identity crisis and was in the process of reverting back to the name of Gilbert Jones.

The journey home I knew nothing about. I awoke to find myself being pulled out of the car by Margaret and pushed by Dr Oaks.

'I'm exhausted,' I remember muttering.

The following morning I woke up with a dreadful headache and a dry mouth. It was some time before I realised that, with the aid of Dr Oaks' flask, I had acquired a magnificent hang-over.

10

THE CAR WAS IN THE GARAGE having a dented panel repaired. The damage had been sustained early one evening while visiting a house on the newly built Charlton Green estate. I'd parked in the road, carelessly leaving the car halfway across a drive belonging to a neighbour of my patient. The neighbour had reversed out of his garage at great speed, omitting to look through his rear window. The resulting collision both repositioned and redesigned my car.

As a result of this slight accident I had been reduced to doing my visits on a borrowed bicycle lent to me by Miss Williams, who had also found me a pair of bicycle clips and a capacious saddle-bag into which I could thrust my bag and a waterproof cape.

Though the bicycle was quite adequate for local calls, it was less suitable for longer journeys. Most weekends I happily spent at home, either looking after the practice or doing odd jobs in the house and garden. But as luck would have it I had arranged to attend a conference in Birmingham the following Saturday.

Scientific conferences today are big business. Doctors, never slow to follow fashions, are avid attenders and rarely a week goes by without there being a conference on some aspect of medical practice somewhere. Most commonly these gatherings are held in Paris, Rome, Brussels, New York, Venice and London, although Vienna, Copenhagen, Washington, Tokyo, Toronto, Athens, Stockholm and Montreal are also popular. The people drinking Pernod in Fouquet's on the Champs Elysées, downing red wine in Florian's in St Mark's Square, or sipping ouzo in the bar of the Grand Bretagne in Athens are almost more likely to be medical delegates than tourists. But each delegate wears a neatly printed name-badge, and at the conclusion of every conference there is at least one important decision to be made – the location of the next meeting.

Naturally when I made arrangements to attend a medical conference it turned out to be in down-to-earth Birmingham rather than exotic Acapulco or the warm Bahamas. Its title, 'The Influence and Importance of Para Medical Disciplines', did at least promise some compensation – although, had I been able to find a sponsor generous enough to provide my travelling expenses, I would have gladly attended a meeting on 'The Importance of Serum Glutaminases in Acromegalic Octogen-arians' if it had been in the Bahamas.

Without my car I had to make the forty-five-mile journey by train. I caught it at half-past eight on Saturday morning. Despite the early hour there were already several hundred passengers installed.

I wandered down it, looking in vain for an empty seat. Every passenger seemed to have commandeered at least two and filled the second up with mackintoshes, hats, newspapers, shopping-bags and briefcases. No traveller appreciates the newcomer who takes the seat next to him, and everyone studiously ignored my enquiring eye.

'Is there anyone sitting here?' I eventually asked an elderly gentleman and his wife who occupied two window-seats. The man did not seem to have heard me. 'Is this seat taken?' I asked, pointing to the one next to him, which bore nothing but a neatly folded copy of *The Times*.

He shook his head and I sat down.

The two of them looked very peaceful and respectable. I thought the gentleman looked rather like a retired school-master. About ten minutes out of the station his wife left us, announcing to her husband that she intended to visit the buffet and purchase a cup of tea. He, a man of obvious discretion, declined her invitation to join her.

She had been gone for no more than a minute when two travellers sitting at the table across the aisle produced a rather scruffy pack of cards.

'Fancy a game?' one of them enquired.

I refused. My neighbour was not so cautious. With only a quick glance in the direction his wife had taken he accepted happily. The result was inevitable. Ten minutes later ten pounds had been transferred from the elderly gentleman's frayed wallet to the much smarter wallet of one of the card-players. I watched in dismay.

The game was in full swing when his wife returned, refreshed. She stood aghast for a moment.

'What are you doing, Henry?' she demanded crossly.

'These gentlemen are teaching me poker, dear,' Henry answered.

'Are you playing for money, Henry?'

'Yes, dear,' replied her hapless husband.

'How much have you lost?' she demanded.

'Ten pounds,' he answered meekly. He went rather pale.

She did not waste time in berating him but turned her attention straight on to the card-player who seemed to be the leader.

'Give my husband back his ten pounds.'

'Now, wait a minute, lady.'

'You give my husband back his ten pounds or I'll pull the communication cord,' screamed the old lady with unexpected fire. She swung her handbag around her head and aimed it at him.

'Hey!' he cried, too late, as the handbag caught him behind his ear. The glass of beer he'd been nursing tipped over and cascaded down my right trouser-leg.

'Right away!' insisted the lady. The old man said nothing but slowly stood up. His wife aimed another blow at the card-player, who opened his wallet and produced his winnings. He handed them over to his assailant.

'I should think so too,' she snapped. 'You ought to be ashamed of yourself. Taking money from such an old man.' With that she took her husband firmly by the arm and led him off down the train. The card-players stared after them, speechless.

Moments later the train drew into Birmingham New Street. I took a taxi to my hotel, not because I felt able to afford such a luxury but because I had no idea at all of the direction and no wish at all to wander around Birmingham on a dreary Saturday morning. The taxi-driver looked at me with pity, accepted me and my small overnight case and deposited us at the correct hotel. He accepted his fare without a word and clearly seemed upset that it had not been accompanied by a generous tip.

'The speaker seems to be suggesting that the use of hypokinase is contraindicated in patients suffering from Von Braun's disease of the splenic flexure,' drawled a man with a thick cigar, scratching his perineum absentmindedly.

'Absolutely right,' confirmed the earnest academic from Toronto. 'I recommend geniprurine for this condition except when there is any underlying hint of incipient myxoedema.'

The cigar-smoker paused for a moment. 'Surely that's jumping out of the therapeutic frying-pan into the pharmacological fire?' he suggested. He looked around when he'd spoken, searching for smiles and nods of appreciation. There were few of either since most of the other delegates had become bored by the long exchange of homilies, clichés and insults which had been going on for nearly three hours.

'That's a very sweeping statement,' the academic argued. 'The drugs in the geniprurine group are well acknowledged to be highly suitable for use in cases where central venous pressure variations are significant.' He polished the hook of his nose with a pale-blue handkerchief. The discussion was really far too technical for me, and I would have had difficulty in keeping awake had I not become aware of the fact that my throat was painfully dry and sore. I was desperate for a drink of water.

'Ah,' said the cigar-smoker, adjusting the bag under his left eyebrow, 'but surely it is as misleading to judge a drug by the character of others in the same group as it is to judge people by the character of others with the same race, religion, profession or circle of friends and acquaintances.'

I wondered if anyone would notice if I crept out of the lecture-theatre. I was sitting in the back row, and the taps and plastic cups in the gentleman's cloakroom were a mere thirty yards away.

The academic speaker had his mind on more important matters.

'That is a calculated insult!' he roared venomously, his face red with rage. 'I must demand an apology!' He turned to the

73

chairman, an inoffensive-looking gentleman wearing a tweed suit and bifocals. 'An apology!' he repeated.

It was then that I noticed the tea-lady had crept into the room, pushing her trolley slowly and gingerly lest its squeaking wheels should disturb the proceedings. I beckoned to her.

'Have you got a glass of water?' I mouthed silently. Leaving her trolley where it was, she tiptoed across to me. I repeated my silent request and pointed to my throat. 'I think I've got a bit of a cold coming,' I added.

The academic speaker, meanwhile, had shot up into the air, opened his mouth, said nothing and sat down again immediately. As mechanically as if he'd been sitting on the other end of a well-oiled see-saw the chairman jumped to his feet and started to clap. The other doctors in the lecture-room followed his example.

'Have two of these, dear,' said the tea-lady, producing a small packet of aspirins from her overall pocket. She hurried back to her trolley and fetched me a cupful of warm water. Obediently I swallowed her advice.

'I must close this discussion period now,' said the chairman with a broad but empty grin as the applause died away. 'I'd like to thank our speakers for their spirited thoughts and for the good-natured way in which they have given us the benefit of their many years of experience.' The academic glowered from behind a water-carafe. The other man sank back into his chair and puffed contentedly on his cigar.

I couldn't help feeling grateful that I'd been treated by the tea-lady rather than by any of my more eminent colleagues. But, like many doctors, I am reluctant to take pills. I know only too well that they can sometimes do more harm than good.

Mrs Barley was one of my first patients in general practice, and when I think of her I still shudder.

She came into the surgery complaining that her bowels were a bit under the weather. Like many patients she treated them rather like naughty children, castigating them if they misbehaved in any way. With reluctance I gave her a bottle of medicine guaranteed by the manufacturers to turn a chronic case of constipation into an acute case of diarrhoea within hours.

She was back the next day clutching the bottle.

'Made me sick, this did,' she complained. 'Brought back some nice stewing steak. Can't be right. Lovely stewing steak, it was.'

I prescribed some pills designed to stop sickness in the time it takes to put away the bucket. Mrs Barley was suspicious and sceptical. She seemed to think she might bring the pills back up, but I told her to persevere.

The pills stopped the sickness without any difficulty, but unfortunately they didn't seem to agree with Mrs Barley. She was soon back. 'I've been taking them for a week now,' she said, 'and the headache is awful.'

'Why didn't you stop taking them when they started to give you a headache?' I asked.

'I had to go on taking them to keep from being sick from that other medicine,' she explained.

'But you were supposed to stop taking that once you'd had your bowels open,' I told her.

'Well, it was so good I thought I'd keep on with it.' She smiled at me. The fruit on her hat wobbled as she coyly shrugged her shoulders. 'I couldn't waste it, could I?'

'You must be sensitive to those pills,' I told her. 'Are you allergic to anything?'

'Only cheap metal jewellery,' she said.

I explained that I had no intention of prescribing that for her, and gave her some enormous white pills to help clear up the headaches. They were so big that I didn't honestly know whether the patient was supposed to swallow them, climb on top of them or eat them with a knife and fork. Mrs Barley didn't seem too sure, either. 'Have they got non-fattening centres?' she asked me.

The headaches went quickly, but she came back complaining of diarrhoea. I gave her a bottle of a new product that the company's representative had compared with cement in its properties. The diarrhoea stopped quickly. Unfortunately she then complained that she'd developed an itch in a personal place. I gave her some cream and pessaries. She also said she couldn't sleep. I gave her sleeping-pills. I was relieved when she didn't appear again for several weeks. I'd half-suspected that the cream for the itch might upset her skin or that the sleeping-tablets might cause constipation.

I managed to get away from the lecture-theatre slightly ahead of the other delegates, who were mobbing the tea-lady. I crawled back to my room and lay down, but the telephone rang before I could get to sleep. It was one of the organisers of the conference, reminding me that there was a free evening ahead and asking if I'd like to join a small party of doctors planning on spending the evening at the cinema.

'I'm not too well,' I told him.

'I'll get someone to call up and see you,' promised the caller.

'It's not serious,' I assured him hastily.

'What's wrong?' asked the caller. 'We have so many specialists around that I'm sure we can find someone to sort you out quickly.'

The trouble with falling ill when you are a doctor is that, even if you only have a headache, some bright fellow will insist on calling in a brain surgeon and having exploratory surgery performed. When looking after each other doctors always feel that they have to be on their best professional behaviour. They order special tests, arrange painful investigations and insist on considering every diagnostic possibility. The doctor who is the doctor always feels that the doctor who is the patient is critically examining his technique. He always does his best to make sure that he gets full marks. Inevitably this often means that the doctor who is the patient has to put up with a lot of unnecessary tests and may well end up feeling far worse than he did before the examination.

'I'll be fine in an hour,' I promised.

'Right,' said the caller. 'We'll meet in the lobby in ninety minutes.'

And so, snuffling, sneezing and coughing, I found myself pacing the streets with a gang of marauding medical men in search of entertainment. Without even looking at the posters outside the cinema I followed the leaders into a dimly lit vestibule. I'd have gone in anywhere to sit down and get warm.

The film was called *The Neighbour's Knickers* and was intended to be an account of swinging life in a northern English town. The commentary was read by a man who sounded as if he usually earned his living reading the football results. Every phrase was carefully weighed and balanced before delivery.

The participants engaged in a series of muscle-numbing callis-
thenics designed for those with insatiable appetites and unlimited patience. They seemed to get us much enjoyment out
of their activities as most people get out of cleaning their teeth
or blowing their noses.

I sneaked out before the end, leaving my colleagues to their
vicarious thrills. When I got back to the hotel my head was
throbbing and I felt unbearably lonely and miserable. I could
have done with at least two more of the tea-lady's aspirin
tablets. Feeling very sorry for myself, I picked up the telephone
and rang Margaret.

'The doctor is away,' she said sleepily. 'Please telephone Dr
Edwards.' She gave the number of Dr Edwards' surgery.

'This is the doctor,' I said.

'Oh, hullo, Dr Edwards.'

'Not him, me.'

'Who?'

'Me.'

'You?'

'Me.'

There was a silence for a moment.

'Is that you, darling?'

I nodded.

'Is that you, darling?' Margaret said again.

'That's right,' I said. 'It's me.'

'I'm sorry,' said Margaret. 'I was asleep.'

'I'm sorry I woke you.'

'That's all right. I'm sorry I didn't recognise your voice.

'Don't keep apologising.'

'I'm sorry.'

Margaret asked me where I'd been and what I'd been doing.
I told her I'd been to a medical film and that it had been very
boring.

'You sound as if you've got a cold coming.'

'I have.'

'That's probably why I didn't recognise your voice. You must
have something for it.'

'I will.'

'Take two aspirin.'

'O.K.'

'Now, promise.'

I promised.

'I put some in your soap-bag,' she said. 'Just in case you needed any.'

She blew me a kiss, I blew her one and we both put our telephones down. Then I found the aspirin tablets, swallowed two and went to bed. It was a double bed and it was very lonely. I realised with some surprise that it was the first time since I'd been married that I'd spent the night away from Margaret.

II

THE GARDEN BEHIND THE SURGERY was mainly designed to satisfy the eyes rather than the stomach. Margaret and I decided that, in order to make ends approximate if not actually meet, we would need to grow our own vegetables. We decided, therefore, to begin by preparing a proper vegetable patch.

And so one Saturday morning I found myself dressed in a thick sweater, old corduroy trousers and wellington boots, and armed with a shiny new spade. We had decided to sacrifice a small area of lawn and a flower-bed. I began by wielding my spade with great enthusiasm. Never having undertaken such a task before, I had no thought of pacing myself. Consequently after twenty minutes or so I was obliged to take time out for refreshments. Margaret, with a slight look of surprise, prepared coffee and biscuits, which she carried out to me on a tray. We sat together and stared gloomily at the small dent my effort had made in the hard ground.

With the coffee all but drunk I was saved from further effort by the telephone.

'It's a Mr Young,' said Margaret, coming out of the house with a piece of paper in her hand. 'He wants you to go and see his wife.'

'Oh dear,' I moaned half-heartedly. 'Now I'll never get the gardening done.'

'Never mind,' she said, handing me the address. 'It'll still be here when you get back.'

Mr and Mrs Young lived in an outlying village. They had a small shop which sold anything and everything imaginable. On the right-hand side was the post office counter where Mrs Young sold stamps, postal orders and savings certificates and gave away gossip, news, information and advice. On the left Mr Young looked after the dried foods, fresh fruit, frozen foods, meat, poultry and farm produce. In the middle Mr and Mrs

Young combined to sell toys, stationery, ironmongery, gardening-tools, newspapers, magazines and books. The shop was known in the other villages as the local Harrods.

'It's the wife,' said Mr Young, leading me through into a small back living-room which was piled high with cardboard boxes of all shapes and sizes. 'She was took bad in the night.'

'I'm sorry to hear that,' I told him, following his footsteps as he carefully made his way towards what looked like a cupboard door. To my surprise it opened to reveal a staircase. Mr Young led the way up.

His wife was lying in bed.

'She's lost 'er mind, Doctor,' said Mr Young, waving a hand in her direction.

'Hullo,' I said to his wife. She said nothing.

'She can't talk,' he said. 'Something 'appened to 'er in the night.'

'Was she all right yesterday evening?' I asked him.

'She were fine yesterday,' he said. 'We 'ad a little celebration yesterday evening on account of our 'aving been married twenty-five years.'

I sat on the edge of the bed. It creaked and sagged uncomfortably.

I took Mrs Young's right arm and held it up above the bed. It felt limp and lifeless. When I let it go it flopped down. Her left arm was much stronger. When I lifted it up it stayed where I'd put it and then was slowly lowered back on to the bedclothes. Her legs were the same. The right leg was weak and powerless, the left seemed quite strong.

'Have you any pain?' I asked her.

She said nothing, but opened her mouth silently. One eye was slightly closed, and her lips were screwed up to one side.

'She's gone and 'ad a turn,' said Mr Young.

'I'm afraid she has,' I agreed.

She looked at me with frightened eyes. She seemed desperate to tell me something. I picked up her left hand and held it in mine.

'Squeeze my hand if you can hear me,' I told her.

She squeezed my hand fiercely until it almost hurt.

'Squeeze it again if you have any pain,' I told her.

Her hand remained quite still.

'Can you understand me?' I asked her. 'Squeeze my hand once if you can.'

Again my hand was squeezed.

I turned to Mr Young. 'Your wife can understand you perfectly well,' I told him, 'but she can't talk to you.'

He looked confused.

'You've had a slight stroke,' I told Mrs Young. 'It's affected your right side and you've lost your speech temporarily.' I looked straight at her. 'Squeeze my hand if you understand that.' She squeezed again.

'I want you to rest,' I told her. 'Stay still and quiet for a day or two.'

She nodded a little.

'I can't promise you anything,' I told her, 'but in a day or two's time I think you'll find that the strength returns to your right arm and leg and you'll be able to speak again. It may take you a while to learn to speak clearly but it'll probably come.'

She stared at me, tears in her eyes.

'Do you understand?' I asked her. She squeezed my hand and smiled very slightly.

'I'm going to go downstairs with Mr Young,' I told her, 'to tell him how to look after you.' She nodded again, almost imperceptibly.

We went downstairs and into the cardboard-box-filled living-room.

'Sit down, Doctor,' said Mr Young, pulling up an empty wooden beer-crate and brushing a few old newspapers from it. I sat down. He overturned a large egg-box and sat down on that.

'What's really the trouble with 'er, then?' he asked me bluntly.

'She's had a stroke, as I said,' I told him. 'Look after her and I think there's a good chance that she'll make a fine recovery.'

'Aren't you sending 'er into 'ospital?' he asked me.

'Not yet,' I told him. 'If I send her into hospital, she'll be amongst strangers and in a strange place. Here at home with you she'll stand a much better chance of getting better quickly.'

'What about pills?' asked Mr Young. The efficacy of some pills in some circumstances has become so well known that many patients believe that all pills are equally efficacious under all circumstances.

'I don't think there's anything that's going to help her,' I told him. 'She needs tender loving care.'

'Could it have been 'er blood-pressure?' asked Mr Young.

I looked at him and a cold feeling spread upwards from my feet. I'd never even taken the poor woman's blood-pressure. I'd been so pleased with myself at finding she could understand me that I'd completely forgotten to do one of the most fundamental examinations in a patient who's had a stroke.

'I'm going to do that now,' I told him. 'I wanted to have a word with you about her first.' I stood up. 'You stay and look after the shop. I'll be down again in a minute.'

I opened the cupboard door again and went back up the narrow staircase. Mrs Young was as we had left her. I took her blood-pressure and examined her carefully this time. Mr Young's presumptive diagnosis was correct. His wife did have high blood-pressure.

'I'm going to give your husband a prescription for you,' I told her. 'I want you to take a pill every morning.' I took Mrs Young's hand again. She squeezed mine in understanding.

Back downstairs I found Mr Young selling two metal coat-hangers and a packet of envelopes to a small boy with a face full of freckles. I waited until he'd finished.

'Her blood-pressure is a little raised,' I told him. I took my pad out of my pocket and wrote out a prescription for some hypotensive drugs. 'I want you to give her one of these every morning.'

He nodded gratefully. 'I thought she ought to 'ave some pills,' he said.

'I'm sorry about my appearance,' I said, as I made my way through the hatch which separated the front of the shop from the back. 'I was in the garden when you phoned.'

'You do a lot of gardening, do you?' he asked.

'Not a lot,' I told him. 'I'm trying to turn a piece of lawn into a vegetable patch.'

' 'Ard work.' He nodded.

'It is indeed.'

'I'll come over with the cultivator, if you like,' he offered. 'We'll clear a third of an acre in 'alf a day.'

'Oh, there isn't anywhere near that much.'

'This afternoon?' he suggested.

'Well, won't that be a bit difficult?' I argued. 'You're wife will need looking after.'

'Sister Watson will be coming in, won't she?' asked Mr Young. 'She's the district nurse.'

'I don't know her,' I admitted.

'Third cottage on the left down the lane. You can't miss it.'

I winced. I do wish the country folk wouldn't say, 'You can't miss it.' I always do.

'I'll certainly go and have a word with her,' I promised.

'Do that,' he said. 'Then I'll come over with the cultivator this afternoon.'

I left the post office and set off down the lane. I passed the first cottage after a mere hundred yards or so and saw the second about half a mile away. I went back for the car. It was just as well I did, for the third cottage was about three and a half miles from the Youngs' shop.

It was small and neat with a thatched roof and walls covered with creeping ivy. On the gate a small sign made out of a piece of bark announced its name, Rose Cottage, while below that a small metal plate bore the warning, 'Beware of the dog.'

I stood outside the gate and called to Sister Watson. There was no reply. I walked a little way along the lane until I could see through the hedge into the back garden. There was no one there.

I was kneeling on the verge with my head pushed through the hedge when I heard a bicycle coming. I withdrew my head and stood up. The rider stopped, leant his machine up against the hedge and walked over to me. Dressed in blue with an old-fashioned helmet perched on top of his round red face he was clearly the village policeman.

'I'm looking for Sister Watson,' I told him, before he could demand an explanation.

'I expect you are, sir,' he said with a slow gruff voice. 'I expect you are.'

'I don't much like dogs, you see,' I told him.

'I don't expect you do, sir.'

'I was hoping I might catch her in the garden.'

'I expect that's right, sir.' The policeman nodded cheerily.

'She has a dog.'

'Has she now, sir?'

'My car's up there,' I told him, pointing to where it stood outside Sister Watson's gate.

'So I see, sir,' said the policeman. He pushed back his helmet and mopped his brow with a huge white handkerchief. I wondered idly why anyone should be perspiring on such a cool day.

'Well, thank you for stopping, officer,' I said, starting back towards the gate.

'Just a moment, if you would be so kind, sir,' the policeman said, taking me by the arm. 'I think we ought to have a word with Sister Watson, don't you?'

'That's right,' I said. 'I do want to speak to her.'

'I expect you do, sir,' he agreed.

He walked back to the gate with me. He bent down, opened it and ushered me through ahead of him. He then banged fiercely on the front door. A minute or two later a small grey-haired woman in a dark-blue uniform opened it.

'Oh, it's you, Arnold,' she said.

'I caught this fellow peering at your marrows,' shouted the policeman. The noise temporarily deafened me.

'I came to ask you to look after Mrs Young,' I told her. 'I'm Doctor Vernon.'

'What's he say, Arnold?' asked the nurse.

'He says he's the doctor, Miss Watson,' said the policeman.

'He's not the doctor, Arnold,' she said. 'Doctor Edwards is much older.'

'I'm not Doctor Edwards,' I said.

'What's he say?' asked Miss Watson.

'He says he's not Doctor Edwards,' shouted Arnold.

'Of course he's not Doctor Edwards,' she scoffed.

'I took over from Dr Oaks when he retired,' I bawled. I could see Arnold taking me back to the village police station.

'Can't stand the man,' said Miss Watson, shaking her head.

'He's retired,' I yelled.

'There's no need to shout,' she said. She turned to Arnold. 'What's he say?'

Eventually we managed to explain the situation. In my turn I learnt that she and Dr Oaks had never seen eye to eye and that he had refused to allow her or any other district nurse to look after any of his patients. But she agreed to take care of Mrs Young. I discovered that if I kept my voice at a certain volume she could hear quite well. The necessary level lay somewhere between a concrete-mixer and a high-performance racing-car engine.

'Where's your dog?' I asked, before I left.

'Dog?'

'It says, "Beware of the dog," on your gate.'

'Oh yes. So it does.'

'Did he die?'

'I've never had a dog,' she said. 'I can't stand dogs.'

'But the sign. . . .'

'I live on my own,' she said. 'The sign was Mr Young's idea several years ago.' She smiled quaintly. 'As a deterrent.' She leant towards me and whispered confidentially, 'I must say, I rather think Mr Young sold it to me because he had a lot of them in stock. I discovered afterwards that just about every cottage in the village had one on the gate.'

I called back at the shop on the way home to tell Mr Young that Sister Watson would be calling round after lunch. In the few moments I spent there he sold me a pot of duck's liver pâté and six metal coathangers.

12

MR YOUNG turned up that afternoon as he had promised, arriving in a small battered van behind which he towed a trailer carrying his cultivator. It was much larger than I had expected and looked more suitable for preparing farmland than vegetable patches. Nevertheless, he assured me that it would be just the thing.

While Margaret and I watched he wheeled the machine down from the trailer and across our garden.

He looked at it and announced, 'About eighteen inches should do it.' He fiddled with his machine and without further delay began to dig away at the grass and soil.

'How kind of him,' whispered Margaret. 'It'll save an awful lot of digging.' We went indoors and left him to it.

He completed work on our patch of land in about half an hour. He put his machine back on to the trailer and knocked on the kitchen door.

'All right, then, Doctor?' he enquired.

'Fine, thank you,' I told him, looking down the garden at the patch of fresh brown earth.

'That'll be ten pounds, Doctor, if you please,' he added.

'Ten pounds?'

'Special price for you,' he murmured confidentially.

I went and fetched a cheque-book.

'Cash, if you don't mind, Doctor,' he said. 'Not that I don't trust you, but in my line of business you can't be too careful.'

'But you know who I am!' I protested.

He winked at me. 'Cash is so much more worthwhile.'

'Ah,' I said, understanding. 'The Inland Revenue.'

'Exactly!' he said. 'Exactly. You've 'it the nail right on the 'ead there, Doctor.'

86

I went and found Margaret sorting out packets of seeds in the living-room.

'Shall we have two packets of lettuce seeds in straight away?' she asked. 'Or shall we keep one for later?'

'Have you got ten pounds?'

'Ten pounds?'

'For Mr Young.'

'Oh,' she said. 'I thought. . . .'

'Yes, that's what I thought.'

Eventually by emptying her purse and all my trouser and jacket pockets we managed to raise £9.55.

'That's all right, Doctor,' said Mr Young. 'You can bring the other forty-five pence out when you come to see the wife.'

It was about two hours later that Margaret first noticed the strange smell.

'That Mr Young certainly gave our garden a good turning over,' she said. 'It smells very rich.'

I sniffed, coughed and agreed with her. The sweet odour of manure was not difficult to detect.

'We'll be able to grow some good vegetables in that,' she said. 'All the books say manure is excellent for them.'

We were congratulating ourselves when the doorbell rang, interrupting our vision of prize-winning beans and gold-medal cabbage.

'I'm from the post office,' said the man at the door.

'Hullo,' said I. 'I'm afraid we gave last Christmas.'

'Got a little problem,' he said, ignoring my witticism, as people always do.

'Oh yes?' said I. 'What can we do to help?'

'Your telephone's out of order,' said the man.

'No, it's all right, thank you,' I told him. 'It was working perfectly well last time it rang.'

'It's not ringing now.'

'No,' I agreed. 'It's not.'

'Report of a faulty service,' he told me.

'Really?' I said. 'I don't think we reported it.'

'Not you,' he replied. 'Another subscriber.'

'Well, you'd better come in and have a look at it,' I told him. I let him in, showed him the telephone in the surgery and went to tell Margaret. She had decided that we'd plant one packet of lettuces and keep one for later in the summer.

'Definitely out of order,' said the engineer, suddenly appearing in the doorway.

'Well, what do we do?' asked I.

'There's nothing wrong with the handset,' he said. He sniffed, screwed up his nose and grimaced.

'What's the matter?' asked Margaret.

'Smell,' he said.

'That's manure,' we both told him at once.

'Been gardening, have you?'

'That's right.' I nodded.

'I'll trace the cable,' he said with another sniff.

He left us, and we began to discuss the relative advantages of growing tomatoes indoors and out of doors. We had made the momentous decision to try some outside and some inside when the engineer returned.

'Spare a minute?' he asked, beckoning.

We obediently followed him outside and down the garden. As we walked we all held our noses tightly.

'The cable's cut,' he said, pointing to a thick curl of black cable which had clearly been severed from some more black cable still underground. 'I'll have to splice it.'

'We had a man in with a cultivator this afternoon,' I told him.

'Always happening,' he nodded. Then he shook his head. 'Very silly.' With his nose still held tightly he sounded as if he'd got a heavy cold.

'Hey!' shouted Margaret, suddenly sinking down to mid-calf in soft soil. I pulled her out with some difficulty.

'Dreadful good smell that,' offered the engineer.

'Look!' cried Margaret, pointing to the hole we'd pulled her out of. It had become a small pond.

'The sewer pipe's fractured,' said the engineer.

'Oh no,' sobbed Margaret. 'It's that Mr Young of yours.' She ran indoors.

'I'll go back to the depot and fetch a crew to get this cable repaired,' said the engineer. 'I'll call the council too, if you like, and get this sewer mended.'

'Thanks very much,' I told him. 'Much appreciated.'

I went slowly back up the garden and into the house. Margaret was upstairs in the bath. I absentmindedly picked up the telephone to ring Mr Young and tell him what his wretched cultivator had done. It was perhaps just as well for us both that I was unable to do so.

13

Mr Young was selling metal coathangers again.

'Very special value,' he insisted as a lady with a large wicker basket, loaded with tins and packets of foodstuffs, pulled a wry face.

'Old stock from the 'olesaler's. We shan't be able to repeat this offer again.'

That turned the odds in his favour, and the customer paid happily for a dozen coathangers.

'Nice to see you, Doctor,' he said to me as she left. 'Come on through.' He led the way.

Then he leant a little closer. 'You 'aven't forgotten that little matter of forty-five pence, 'ave you, Doctor?' he asked in a conspiratorial whisper.

'Not at all,' I told him. 'Can I have a word with you about it when I come down?'

'Certainly, Doctor. I'll be 'ere.'

Mrs Young was lying in bed just as she had been when I'd last seen her two days before.

'Hullo!' I said. 'How are you doing?'

'I ... can ... talk ... a ... little ... thank ... you ... Doctor,' she said, very slowly and deliberately.

'That's wonderful!' I exclaimed with genuine delight. I sat down on the edge of her bed again.

'I ... can ... move ... my ... arm ... and ... leg ... a ... little,' she said, moving her previously paralysed arm an inch or two off the bedclothes.

'That's splendid,' I told her. 'You must move it as much as you possibly can now. The more you use it, the quicker it will grow strong again.'

'I ... tried ... to ... get ... up ... this ... morning,' she told me, 'but ... I ... was ... very ... dizzy.'

'What happened?' I asked her.

'I . . . nearly . . . fell . . . over.'

'I'll take your blood-pressure again,' I told her. I took out the sphygmomanometer and wrapped the cuff around her upper arm. I took her blood-pressure twice, I was so surprised by the amount it had fallen.

'I'm afraid it's dropped too much,' I told her. 'We'll have to stop your pills!'

She looked slightly embarrassed.

'What's the matter?' I asked her.

'The . . . pills,' she said. 'I'm . . . sorry.'

'Don't you be sorry!' I laughed. '*I'm* sorry they were too powerful for you. We'll try you without anything for a day or two and then check it again.'

I put my sphygmomanometer away. Then I shook hands with her, reassured her that she should do as much as she could, and made my way back downstairs. In the shop Mr Young was busy serving a gentleman in a tweed suit and fishing-hat who'd come in for some tobacco. This time he failed in his attempts to unload more metal coathangers.

'Your wife has made a great recovery,' I told him when the fisherman had finally left.

'She's a little better,' he conceded, 'but she's a bit flat.' He led me back into the living-room and we pulled up our respective boxes again. ' 'Er get-up-and-go 'as got up and gone.'

'She's been a bit dizzy,' I agreed. 'I'm afraid those pills I gave her proved a little too strong for her.'

'Ah,' said Mr Young.

'I've stopped them,' I told him.

'Stopped them altogether?'

I nodded.

'Is that wise?'

'Well, I think so,' I told him, aggrieved at having my decision challenged so openly.

'She's been taking three a day,' he said.

'Three a day!' I cried. 'She's only supposed to be on one a day, I'm sure. Where's the bottle?'

He handed it to me from behind a clock on the mantelpiece.

'There you are,' I told him. ' "One every morning".'

'Well,' he said, 'I thought if she was going to get better with one a day she ought to get better three times as quickly on three a day.'

'Mr Young,' I said, very slowly and deliberately, 'you could have killed your wife.'

He went very white and began to bluster.

'I need 'er back in the shop,' he protested. 'I can't look after it all by myself.'

'If you want her to get better, then do what I suggest,' I told him. 'And, if you haven't got any faith in my abilities as a doctor, then I'd rather you found a doctor in whom you do.'

He sniffed and scratched the side of his head.

'You must see what I mean,' I said, feeling rather guilty after my outburst.

'Yes, Doctor,' he muttered with a half-embarrassed grin. 'I'm sorry.'

'Right,' I said, 'I'll go back upstairs and tell her to carry on taking the tablets as I originally instructed.' I paused as I headed for the cupboard door. 'How many has she taken today?'

'Just the one this morning,' he said. 'That's the honest truth, Doctor.'

'I hope it is.' I went back upstairs and spoke to Mrs Young. She blushed again and haltingly apologised.

'Forget it,' I told her. 'But do as I've asked, will you?'

She promised that she would.

I then went back downstairs yet again. 'Will you be calling back?' Mr Young asked as he followed me out.

'Has Sister Watson been in?'

'Oh yes,' he said, 'she comes twice a day.'

'Then I'll be back in two days,' I told him. 'Unless there's been any change. You must ring me if there are any problems at all.'

'Fine,' he said. 'Thank you, Doctor. I'm sorry about the pills.'

I waved my hand.

'You 'aven't, er, forgotten the forty-five pence, 'ave you, Doctor?' he called, as I opened the front door.

'I'm glad you reminded me about that,' I said. I took my hand off the door-handle and stepped back into the shop. He smiled expectantly.

I told him what had happened.

'Oh deary me,' he said. 'Is everything sorted out?'

'It is now,' I told him.

'You should have given me a call before,' he said. 'I'd have come and put it all right for you.'

'I would have,' I told him, 'but unfortunately the telephone was out of order and I couldn't. The post office had to transfer all our calls to Miss Williams at home and she had to come round and give me messages.'

'Oh deary me,' he said again. 'I must have gone down much too deep.'

'I think that must have been it,' I agreed.

'I did say eighteen inches, didn't I?'

I nodded.

'They put sewage pipes and telephone cables much deeper than that.'

'I hope they do.'

'Still,' he said. 'You did have a bit of trouble, didn't you?'

I agreed.

'Then I'll not charge you any extra,' he said. 'I dug too deep – that usually costs more.'

'I beg your pardon?' I could hardly believe my ears.

'We'll just settle the forty-five pence,' he said, 'and call it quits.'

I know when I'm beaten. I handed him the money and left.

14

'THERE'S A PATIENT in the waiting-room I think you ought to
see straight away,' said Miss Williams, slipping into the surgery as the previous patient slipped out.

'Right,' I said, happy as always to accept her experienced and
expert advice. 'Send him in.'

'It's dear old Mr Campion,' she said, disappearing again.

Mr Campion's gnarled right arm was badly gashed and,
although it was roughly bound with a piece of once white
cloth, blood was still dripping from the cut.

'How did you do that?' I asked him, sitting him down and
unwrapping the wounded limb.

'Scythe,' said Mr Campion. 'Darned fool thing to do.' He
shook his head in disgust as I finally unveiled it. 'I was cutting
a bit of rough grass behind the cow shed.'

'How did you get to the surgery?' I asked him.

'Come up on my bicycle,' he told me. 'It's only three or four
miles.'

I began to swab the wound with a piece of alcohol-soaked
cotton-wool. 'You rode your bicycle here with that cut in your
arm?' I asked in amazement.

'There ain't no buses at this time of day.'

'How old are you, Mr Campion?'

'Ninety-one,' came the proud reply.

'You still work on a farm?'

'Only five days a week.'

I finished cleaning up the wound and decided to put a few
stitches in it.

'Haven't you ever thought of retiring?' I asked him.

'What would I want to retire for?' he asked. 'I don't want
to spend my last days doing nothing. I want to wear out, not
rust out.'

'Well, you'll wear yourself out pretty quickly if you keep
taking pieces out of yourself like this,' I told him.

'I ain't got nothing to save myself for,' he grinned.

I had to concentrate for a few minutes while putting in the stitches. When I'd finished I gave him a tetanus injection.

'Have you a little bandage, Doctor?' he asked.

'You don't really need a bandage on it.'

'I don't want to get it dirty.'

'You're not going back to work, are you?' I asked, astonished.

'That grass ain't going to get any shorter if I don't cut it.'

'Is there anyone who can take you back to the farm?' I asked, having bandaged the arm. 'Or can I give you a lift out there?'

'I've got my bicycle, thank you, Doctor,' he replied.

I escorted him to the door and waved as he set off slowly up the road. With a shout I reminded him to return in a week to have the stitches removed.

It was ten days later while cutting the back lawn that I suddenly remembered he had never returned to have his wound checked or stitches taken out. I left the grass half-shorn, went into the surgery and found his notes. The address they bore was Hell's End Cottage, Waverley Lane. I'd never heard of the place, and studying a large-scale map of the area told me nothing. I telephoned the local ambulance station. They had never heard of it, either. I then tried the police station and the post office. No one at either of these two establishments could help me.

'Try the Reverend Dewhurst,' suggested the police station sergeant. 'I do hear that he's writing a history of the town.'

I waited another day, hoping that Mr Campion would turn up at the surgery of his accord, but when there was still no sign of him I decided to follow the sergeant's advice.

The vicarage was fairly easy to find. Like so many vicarages this one was far larger than was practical or necessary, having been built in the days when clergymen were relatively wealthy, certainly widely respected and able to employ a fair number of servants to keep their homes and families in good order and repair. Today's incumbent had clearly long since abandoned all hope of maintaining the whole place properly. The garden was slightly overgrown and the house itself would have provided a small building firm with plenty of work for a couple of years.

I pressed the doorbell several times but got no reply. Only

then did I suspect that it might not be working. My suspicions were justified when a rat-a-tat on the handsome brass knocker produced an immediate response.

'I'm looking for the vicar,' I told the homely-looking soul who opened the door. She wore her hair in a delightfully neat old-fashioned bun.

'So am I,' came the unexpected reply.

'Where do you think we might find him?' I asked.

'Heaven knows,' she answered, with undoubted justification. 'Is he out?' I asked.

'I think he said he was going into the garden,' she replied, 'but I've been calling him for twenty minutes – his lunch is ready.'

'Can I wander round and look for him?'

'Please do. If you find him, you might tell him his lunch is spoiling.'

I discovered the vicar squatting on a sawn-off tree-stump amongst a mass of head-high daisies, just in bloom.

'Hullo there!' I called cheerily. 'Can I have a word with you?'

'Sh!' He held a finger to his lips. 'Look!'

He pointed to a spot about three yards away where a black-bird was feeding worms to an enormous fledgling.

'What on earth is it?' I asked, in a whisper.

'It's a cuckoo. That poor blackbird has been looking after it for weeks now.' He chuckled. 'Poor wretch hardly knows what's happened to him.'

We watched the two birds for a few minutes before eventually they both hopped away in search of further food supplies. 'Your lunch is spoiling,' I told the vicar when he had finally lost sight of them.

'You're not the new choirboy, are you?' he asked suddenly.

'No,' I admitted. I told him my name.

'Oh yes,' nodded the vicar, suddenly remembering me. He blushed. 'I'm still waiting to hear from the plastic surgeon.'

'I've got a bit of a problem,' I said, and explained why I had come. 'There doesn't seem to be a Waverley Lane in the town.'

'Ah, no, indeed,' he said. 'There was but there isn't. It used to be a pleasant country lane, but about twenty years ago a builder got planning permission to turn it into part of a housing estate. Now it's called Ackles Estate after Councillor Ackles who used to be mayor at one time.'

'Well, what happened to Hell's End Cottage?' I asked.

He shook his head sadly. 'That was a lovely old cottage. Oak beams and thatched roof.' He stopped to pick a couple of wild poppies. 'But it was knocked down when they started building.'

'Oh,' said I, 'then that's the end of my search for Mr Campion.'

'You're not looking for old Ebenezer Campion, are you?'

'Tanned old man, nearly bald, ninety?'

'That's Ebenezer!' cried the vicar. 'Why didn't you say you were looking for him? He's been a great help to me. I'm writing a history of the town and he's been here longer than anyone alive.'

'Where can I find him?'

'He's got a cottage on the farm behind the Ackles Estate,' the vicar said. He gave me detailed instructions on how to get there. I thanked him, reminded him about his lunch and hurried off, leaving him studying a pair of blue tits playing around an old tree-stump.

Ebenezer Campion answered the door himself when I called.

'I half-expected to find you out,' I told him as he led me into his tiny cottage.

'I've not been well,' he said, in explanation rather than complaint. He did look ill, much weaker than when I'd seen him before.

'I've come to get those stitches out.'

'Oh, I took them out,' he told me.

'Took them out?' Used to patients who are reluctant to treat their own colds I was surprised to find someone happy to perform an operation, albeit a minor one, himself.

'Nicked them with a razor,' he explained. He pulled up his shirt-sleeve and showed me the healing scar.

'Well, what's been keeping you in, then?' I asked him.

'Born too soon,' he said enigmatically.

'Come on, now,' I told him firmly. 'What's been the trouble?'

'I've been a bit off colour,' he admitted with some reluctance.

'Any pain?'

'A little,' he confessed. 'Just a little.'

'Get your things off. Let me have a look at you.'

'There's no need for that,' he protested. 'Give me a script for a tonic.'

'Let's have a look at you.'

The old man reluctantly pulled open his jacket, waistcoat, shirt and vest to reveal a small triangle of white skin.

'That's no good,' I told him. 'Take them off.'

Very slowly he did so.

'You've lost a lot of weight, haven't you?' I said, quite shocked to see how thin he was.

'A bit,' he admitted.

'Been sick?'

'A bit.'

'You've not been eating much, have you?'

'Not much.' He rubbed his tanned brown hands across his chest. The contrast to his white skin was stark.

It didn't take long to discover that he was beyond my help. He had a mass in his abdomen which I could easily feel. I felt fairly certain that he had a carcinoma of the stomach.

'It's not too good, is it, Doctor?' he asked.

I looked at him. He looked back at me unblinkingly.

'I've been getting weaker for months,' he told me quietly. 'I've never cut myself with a scythe before.'

'It's not too good,' I said quietly.

'I don't want to go into hospital,' he said. 'I don't want to die with bits and pieces stuck into me and people all around me. I like my quiet.'

I nodded. I couldn't think of anything to say. If I live to be a general practitioner for another fifty years, I doubt if I'll ever know what to say to people like Mr Campion.

'Let me stay here, then, will you, Doctor?'

'All right,' I agreed.

'I can manage by myself,' he insisted. 'I don't eat much. Just a little tea and some stew now and then.'

'I'll pop in tomorrow,' I told him.

'It's been a good life, you know. I've been as fit as a damned butcher's dog most of it,' he grinned.

I left, assuring him again that I wouldn't send him into hospital.

Five days later he died. He made no more fuss about dying than he had about living, but did it quietly and with dignity.

15

IT WAS NOT DIFFICULT to find No. 43 Bilberry Rise. Half a
dozen police cars, all complete with illuminated signs and flashing lamps, were parked along the kerbside directly outside it.
A crowd of people, large enough to celebrate the visit of a pop
star with a significant reputation, were kept at bay by policemen in uniform holding lengths of rope.

I parked sixty or seventy yards away from the house and
walked back through the crowd. This was not easy since most
of the people I struggled past seemed to think I was simply
trying to obtain a better vantage-point.

'Who do you think you're pushing?' demanded a monster
of a man who wore a pair of brown corduroy trousers and a
string vest, as I attempted to squeeze past him.

'There's eggs in that basket,' complained an elderly woman
in a blue plastic mac and transparent rain-hood.

Only when I finally reached the rope did I breathe easily. I
would never have guessed that anything could have been fascinating enough to drag so many people from their Sunday
lunch.

The policeman guarding the small rectangle of pavement
and grass in front of the house examined me with suspicion.
Even when I'd explained who I was he still seemed convinced
that I was a reporter of some kind.

'*I* don't even know what I'm doing here,' I told him. 'I just
got a telephone call from the police station asking me to get
here as soon as I could.'

'Give you a bit of an appetite, then,' he said with a wink.
He let me under the rope. The front door was guarded by
another policeman who was more reluctant to allow me
through; it wasn't until I'd opened the black bag I'd dragged
along with me and shown him the absence of cameras and the

presence of stethoscope and sphygmomanometer that he was convinced. He opened the door and let me into the hall.

I have never seen so many people in a small terraced house. In contrast to those outside most of the policemen in the house were out of uniform.

'Doctor?' asked a man with a beard and a tape-recorder.

I nodded.

'Sergeant Grant,' he said. 'I'll take you in to Detective Inspector Dugdale.'

'Doctor?' said a tall well-dressed man with a toothbrush moustache.

I nodded.

'Detective Inspector Dugdale,' he said.

I shook his outstretched hand.

'I'd like you to meet Detective Chief Superintendent Pulpit of the Regional Serious Crimes Squad,' said Inspector Dugdale reverentially.

Chief Superintendent Pulpit, with his fiery red nose, slightly bloodshot eyes and overhanging abdomen, looked more like a publican than a detective. He, too, shook my hand.

'Sorry to drag you away from your Sunday lunch, Doctor,' he said. 'Won't keep you long.'

I muttered some pleasantry.

'It's about a body,' he went on. 'Just want you to certify it for us. No need to do anything more,' he said. 'We've got a forensic pathologist coming along to take a look but we can't move the body until a doctor's had a look. Detective Inspector Dugdale will take you to it.'

With that he decided our meeting was over, and turned away to examine a sheaf of notes offered him by yet another subordinate.

'Sergeant Grant,' said Inspector Dugdale. 'Will you take the doctor to the body?'

Sergeant Grant, who'd been hovering on the outskirts of the conversation, stepped forward, took me by the elbow and steered me skilfully through a small army of technicians and investigating officers who seemed to be making notes about every item of furniture in the house.

'Here you are,' he said finally, coming to a halt at the back door. Over the garden fence I could see several rows of faces peering blankly at me. The sergeant pointed to a dustbin. A large canvas sheet, being fastened on to several poles by a tall red-haired policeman, shielded it from public view.

'Don't touch anything you don't have to touch,' he said, lifting the dustbin lid with a handkerchief wrapped round his hand.

I peered inside, not knowing quite what to expect. I could see nothing but a pile of potato peelings and empty tins, and a cornflake box advertising at a remarkably low price a rubber dinghy complete with oars, lifebelts and distress flares.

'Just here,' said the sergeant, delicately lifting out two strands of peel. That movement exposed what looked like an over-ripe sausage. Closer examination, with eyes and nose, revealed that it was in fact a human finger. A gold ring encircled the middle of it. I took a pair of rubber gloves from my black bag and reached gingerly into the dustbin. Moving an empty baked-beans tin I could see that the hand was attached to an arm but that the arm didn't seem to be attached to anything.

'All right, Doc?' asked the sergeant.

'It seems human,' I agreed. 'Is there any more?'

'We think it's all there,' he said.

I moved an empty sardine tin and revealed a foot. Lifting a yoghurt carton exposed another hand.

'Human?' he asked.

'I think so,' I said. Sunday lunch seemed a long way away.

'Just for the record,' he said, 'if you could dictate a short statement.' I dictated something to the effect that at Sunday lunchtime I had certified as being human and dead parts of a body in a dustbin. Then the sergeant escorted me back to the front door. The officers in the house were still busy.

'Any leads?' I whispered before I finally left.

'Oh, we know who did it,' said the sergeant. 'He's confessed.'

'Who?'

'Husband,' he whispered.

'Why all the fuss, then?' I whispered back.

'Oh, we don't get many murders round here,' he explained.

Outside the crowd of spectators was, if anything, thicker than before.

I'd been invited to act as Temporary Police Surgeon for the local force after the previous holder of the office, who had been Official Police Surgeon for the county, had retired prematurely and with very little notice after inheriting a small but pleasing fortune from a grateful patient.

The appointment added a small retainer to my annual income and each time I was called for advice, medical aid or opinion I received an additional fee. The job was not well paid, but it seemed likely that with its help I would be able to purchase a newer and more reliable motor car in the not too distant future.

One of my responsibilities was looking after the health of the local police. Since policemen and policewomen are, by and large, healthy specimens this was not particularly arduous. In fact, in the first three months I had only two problems to deal with.

The first concerned W.P.C. Jenny Ralston, who complained that every time she wore plain clothes she had a bad back. She herself felt that perhaps the dark-blue tunic of her uniform provided her with more support. A little detective work unearthed a more likely explanation. When wearing her official uniform W.P.C. Ralston wore black low-heeled shoes. When in her own clothes she wore much more fashionable but less orthopaedically desirable platform-soled shoes. These had clearly led to the development of the W.P.C.'s bad back. By the simple expedient of suggesting that she abandon her fashionable aspirations in the interests of her spine I managed to cure her.

The second problem was more serious. Sergeant Martin came to surgery complaining of a number of different symptoms. He was, he said, losing weight. He also mentioned various strange abdominal pains and said he had a problem with his bladder.

'It's most embarrassing,' he told me. 'If I'm on foot patrol, I have to keep popping into the public lavatories. If I'm on patrol in a car, the chap I'm with thinks I'm funny if I keep asking him to stop or go back to the station.'

'Have you noticed that you're thirsty a great deal?' I asked.

He leant across the desk. 'Funny you should say that,' he confided. 'I'm always thirsty. Drink gallons of water every day.'

I asked him to go to the lavatory and pass a specimen of urine for me to test. Once I had that, it wasn't difficult to make the diagnosis. Sergeant Martin had diabetes mellitus.

'Diabetes,' he said in horror when I told him. 'It can't be.'

'I'm afraid it is,' I said.

'Oh dear,' he said, settling down on a chair with a great sigh of despair.

'About two people in every hundred have diabetes,' I told him in an attempt at reassurance. 'Most of them live very normal lives.'

'I appreciate that.'

'Well, then?'

'It's not the diabetes I'm worried about.'

'Well, what on earth is it?' I asked, puzzled.

'My job,' he said. 'I've been a policeman all my life.'

'Well, you won't have to leave the force, will you?' I asked him, aghast.

'They'll let me stay in,' he said, 'but they'll give me a desk job. I can't stand desk work.'

'Well, do they have to know?'

He looked at me as if I'd suggested that we rob a train or bank together.

'What?' he whispered.

'Do they have to know you've got diabetes?'

'Well . . .,' he began. 'I'm not sure.'

'I shan't tell them,' I assured him.

'You won't?'

'Of course not,' I said. 'Your medical condition concerns you and me and no one else.'

'Well, perhaps they needn't know,' he said with the beginnings of a smile. 'Do I have to go into hospital?'

'I don't think so,' I told him. 'I'll want you to get some tests done and see a specialist, but there won't be any need for you actually to go into hospital.'

His condition improved appreciably under treatment with insulin, and when I saw him a week or two later he was quite contented. I had a telephone call from a superintendent at the local station who wanted to know what was wrong with the sergeant, but I muttered something about his being much better and my not being able to give precise details about a patient's condition. The superintendent seemed satisfied. If he suspected anything serious, he was prepared to turn a blind eye.

Most of my work for the police was done at the local police station. There was, for example, the burglar who had hurt his back climbing out through a bathroom window on the first floor of a block of flats. He insisted, however, that his back had been made worse by ill treatment at the hands of the police. Although my examination revealed nothing more than a little bruising, it is impossible to be absolutely certain that there is no bone injury when a patient complains of a back pain. My patient complained that he couldn't even stand up, let alone walk.

I was about to arrange for an ambulance to come and take the prisoner along to the local hospital X-ray department under escort when Detective Inspector Dugdale appeared.

'Get up, you lousy layabout!' he screamed. He frightened me too.

The prisoner jumped to his feet in an instant, apparently cured.

Even more potentially embarrassing was the man who, arrested for drunken driving and brought to the police station to have a blood sample taken, insisted that I take it from his penis.

'I usually take blood from the arm,' I pointed out.

'Take it from me prick,' insisted the drunk, pointing to his crotch, 'or not at all.'

I was stymied. This time it was Sergeant Martin who came to my rescue.

'You want the doctor to take the blood sample from your penis, do you?' he said, taking a piece of paper from a drawer.

'Tha'ss right,' nodded the drunk.

'Fine,' said Sergeant Martin. 'You'll just have to sign this.'

'Wha'ss that?'

'Oh, just a clearance form,' said the sergeant. 'Sometimes when the doctor takes blood from a penis it will shrivel up and fall off. You have to sign to say you don't mind if that happens.'

The drunk began feverishly rolling up his sleeve.

16

THE TWO TEAMS OF WORKMEN arrived within five minutes of one another. The first team came in a small lorry and they brought with them a pneumatic drill, a small generator, a nice variety of picks, a shovel and a large wooden hut which they erected outside the surgery seconds after their arrival and in front of which they immediately positioned a large oil-drum with holes drilled in the sides of it. They filled this with coke, set fire to it and then balanced an ancient blackened kettle on top.

The second team also came in a small lorry but they brought with them two step-ladders, a dozen planks, a variety of scaffolding poles, several large cans of green paint, a bucketful of old brushes and a neat modern gas-stove on top of which they balanced an ancient blackened kettle.

I was standing in the front garden when they arrived, trying as usual to decide which plants were weeds and which were not. I watched them with curiosity. Having settled down, they watched each other with caution, like two opposing armies before a big battle. They gathered in silent semi-circles behind their bubbling kettles, studied their newspapers without much obvious interest and stared at each other.

The kettles having been boiled, the tea having been made and drunk, two men in corduroy trousers, wellingtons and donkey jackets took pickaxes to attack the large concrete grit-bin which stands just outside the surgery and which seems to serve little useful purpose since the road in which the surgery is situated is as flat as a road can be.

Before the first pickaxe could strike two men from the opposing camp rushed to the rescue.

'Hey!' they cried in musical unison. 'Stop that!'

The pickaxe wielding workmen halted in midswing and then slowly and clumsily lowered their weapons to the ground.

'We've got to paint that bin green,' protested one of the opposing workmen.

'No,' insisted the others. 'It's got to be demolished.'

The argument had attracted the attention of the rest. Soon they were all gathered around the coke-burning oil-drum drinking tea again. I left them and returned indoors. Surgery was due to start.

The ways of the local authority are not easy to understand. Living in the surgery it was sometimes easy to forget that we were much luckier than most of our patients whose homes belonged to or were at the mercy of the Council.

Some patients, like Mr and Mrs Willow found their lives interfered with through absolutely no fault of their own. They lived in an old three-room cottage which had once stood alone surrounded by fields and meadows. As the century progressed the fields and meadows had been replaced by houses and schools, the trees and streams by lamp-posts and roads, and the peace and quiet by suburban buzz. Despite all these changes Mr and Mrs Willow had stayed on in their cottage, which stood out dramatically amidst the neat rows of town houses.

It had once been owned by a farmer. When he had sold his land to property developers the cottage had been sold too. The developers had been anxious to remove Mr and Mrs Willow from their home, but before they could do so they had gone bankrupt. The local authority had taken over the company and with it the cottage. They, too, had been anxious to move their tenants to another home and to build a small group of maisonettes on the site.

'They want us to go and live in a block of flats for old people,' Mr Willow told me as I examined his right leg one day.

'You've got a bit of arthritis here,' I told him.

'What do we want to live in a block of flats for?' he demanded. 'We like our cottage. What do we want a bathroom for?'

I rolled his trouser-leg back down.

'Arthritis?' said he, looking down. 'Why've I got that, then?'

'It comes to us all with age.'

'What about this one?' he asked, patting his left leg.

'Seems all right.'

'It's as old as the other,' he insisted.

'You might like it,' I suggested, 'with lots of people of your own age.'

'I hate old people,' he snapped. 'They never seem to have any fun.' He smoothed his trouser-leg reflectively. 'I like children,' he smiled.

'They can't make you move, can they?'

He nodded unhappily. 'They say our cottage isn't fit for human habitation. But we've lived in it for fifty years.' He poked a finger in his left ear. 'You can't beat the bureaucrats,' he said sadly. 'My wife won't go downstairs of a morning until I've been to make sure there aren't any buff envelopes on the mat.'

He scratched his other ear. 'My missus isn't as bright as she was,' he said. 'She gets all confused when we go to our Hilda's and watch the telly. She can't understand what them people in the advertisements have got to do with the programme. I don't think she'd make it much longer if we had to move out.'

I saw Mr and Mrs Willow several times and they both grew gradually more and more depressed as it became clear that they were not going to be able to fight off the local authority's attempts to move them to a council flat. Eventually they became so depressed that I prescribed drugs for them both.

As it happened they never did go. They were found dead together by the bailiffs who came to move them out. They had taken all the antidepressant pills I'd prescribed and, although that in itself would not have proved fatal, they had both drifted into unconsciousness and become incontinent. Their one modern luxury was an electric blanket which they had left switched on. They'd been electrocuted and died without regaining consciousness. The coroner had recorded a verdict of accidental death; but the local authority should perhaps have taken the blame.

Most of the town's Irish Catholic community were on another doctor's list. But the O'Malleys were on mine. They lived in a prefabricated bungalow that had been erected during the Second World War as part of a national attempt to alleviate the chronic housing shortage as quickly and cheaply as possible. It had been intended to last for five years, but a quarter of a century later it was still occupied and there seemed little chance that it would be available for demolition at any time in the foreseeable future.

Mr O'Malley had once worked as a plumber's mate, but for fifteen of his thirty-five years he had lived on the unearned income provided by the D.H.S.S. He, his wife, and their four children were on the Council's housing list but seemed destined to remain in their bungalow indefinitely.

I first met them when I was working as assistant to Dr Oaks. I remember our first confrontation well. I'd been called at about half-past one in the morning by Mr O'Malley, who was clearly metabolising a considerable amount of alcohol.

'It's the baby, Doc,' he said when he'd finally managed to push his change into the coin-box.

Try as I might, I was quite unable to get any further information from him. I pulled on my clothes and set off into the night. I knew roughly where the O'Malleys lived – I'd been to the estate before – but I had no idea which particular bungalow was theirs. I had, therefore, asked him to turn on a light to guide me through the night.

When I arrived on the estate there were several lights in view and I called at each house in turn. There were no numbers on any of the houses and no one seemed to have any idea of their neighbours' identity. After three-quarters of an hour I returned home soaked to the skin without having found the baby. I stayed awake all night worrying about what I'd say to the coroner and the press when it was found dead the next morning.

With the aid of Dr Oaks I did eventually find the right bungalow in daylight.

'Oh, you needn't have bothered coming,' said Mrs O'Malley, a baby hanging on to her milk-heavy breast. 'The baby's fine now.'

'Your husband seemed worried.'

'He always worries,' she said. 'She'd woken up and he wanted you to help put her to sleep.'

I said nothing. Dr Oaks raised a quizzical eyebrow.

'I told him he shouldn't have called you,' she said in her own defence.

'He said he'd leave a light on so that I could find the right bungalow,' I went on.

'Oh, I put the light out so that you'd know we didn't need you,' she said with a kind smile. 'I didn't want you driving around all night or getting wet.'

After that memorable occasion I met the O'Malleys frequently until I got to know them and their bungalow well. Their home was grubby and poorly looked after, adorned only by a variety of elaborate crucifixes, and I suspect that even if they had been allocated a new one they would within a fairly short time have converted it into a slum ready for demolition.

My relationship with them became stronger when I managed to help Mrs O'Malley lose some weight. When I first took over her medical care she weighed sixteen stone. She came to see me and asked if she could go on the Pill.

'I don't want any more,' she said defiantly. 'And it's not the Pope that has to feed them.'

I weighed her, took her blood-pressure and told her that I'd prescribe the contraceptive pill for her on condition that she lost some weight.

'What about the Pill, though?' she insisted as I gave her a diet sheet and instructed her for the fourth time in the rudiments of dieting.

'I'll give you a prescription for a month,' I told her. 'You must come back and see me again then and, if you've lost some weight, I'll give you another month's supply.'

To my surprise she took the blackmail well and over the next six months lost four stone.

Then she heard that the Council would rehouse her and her family if she had another child. Five children are apparently too many for a prefabricated bungalow, although four are not.

She stopped taking the Pill, forgot about dieting, had her fifth and put her four stone back on again. She, her husband and all their children were then rehoused in a seventeenth-floor council flat. Three weeks later they were back squatting in their bungalow, which had been half-destroyed by vandals and which was at long last scheduled for demolition.

When I'd finished surgery the workmen had clearly come to some agreement. They were all drinking a celebratory cup of tea.

'Well, what's the decision?' I asked one of the pickaxe-wielders, as I prepared to have another look at the garden.

'They're going to paint the damned thing,' he replied, 'and then we're going to knock it down.'

17

'IVAGOTABITABADABACKA,' complained Mr Pirelli, limping into the surgery.

I looked at him and waved him to the chair. 'You've a what?' I asked.

'Ivagotabitabadabacka,' he repeated slightly louder.

Slowly I translated the complaint into more comprehensible form. 'You've got a bad back?' I asked.

'Datsaita!' He smiled.

We smiled at each other and both nodded.

'How long have you had a bad back?' I asked him, speaking as slowly and clearly as I could.

'Today.'

'Just today?'

'Today,' he agreed. 'Yesterday and today.'

'You've had a bad back for two days?' I said, reaching for my pen and beginning to write his notes.

'Datsaitaivagotabitabadabackatoday!' cried Mr Pirelli, who seemed to understand my English more easily than I understood his.

'Have you ever had back pain before?'

'No,' came the reply. 'Justatoday.'

I looked at the pile of people's notes stacked on my desk. There were another twenty patients sitting in the waiting-room.

'Rest!' I told him. 'Rest! O.K.'

He looked at me, clearly puzzled. 'Rest O.K.' He nodded.

'Rest a week,' I added.

'No,' he said. 'Rest O.K.'

'Yes,' I struggled on bravely. 'Rest for a week. O.K.'

He stared at me silently for several moments. Very slowly a smile of understanding began to creep across his face.

'Aha!' He grinned. 'Resta.'

'Resta.' I nodded back at him. 'Restaweek. O.K.?'

'Notarest,' he said, shaking his head and holding up his left hand. With his right forefinger he pointed to his left wrist. 'Notarest.'

'Wrist!' I exclaimed. 'No, not your wrist.'

'Rest O.K.,' he assured me. 'Notaweaka.'

'Good.' I smiled back at him. 'I'm glad your wrist is O.K. You must rest for a week.' I gazed at the pile of records again and stood up. Mr Pirelli stood up too, grimacing as he unfolded.

'Nota,' he said. 'Nota fora SOCIAL SECURITY.' He shouted the last two words and said them very slowly and clearly.

I nodded, writing out the necessary certificate and handing it to him.

'Restaweek,' he said, limping towards the surgery door.

'Restaweek,' I agreed.

Communicating with patients is not always easy. There are a thousand potential pitfalls for the doctor who enters general practice. Some patients do not mean what they say, others do not say what they mean. Many cannot say what they want to say and many more cannot understand what is said to them, although they will profess understanding. And the English language can cause the unwary to wander from one disaster to another purely and simply because of misunderstanding due to nationality, class or dialect.

To add to the confusion inevitable in any moderately cosmopolitan community there are the further confusions caused by colourful phrases and euphemisms which vary a great deal from area to area and even from family to family. The phrases, 'a frog in the throat', 'a flea in his ear', 'water on the knee' and 'butterflies in his stomach' are fairly well known to those brought up on the English language, but there are others, far less well known, which can, either by their being used or by their not being used, cause untold problems. Many people favour expressions to describe bodily functions which mean nothing at all to others born in the same town, let alone abroad. It is rare for any patient to talk about urinating or micturating. Most will talk of passing water, spending a penny, piddling, tiddling, going to see a man about a dog, doing a number one, pissing or going for a wee-wee. A woman's monthly period is described variously as a curse, a visitor or a time of the month, and its absence may denote either being in the pudding club or having a bun in the oven. When angry a man will describe himself as being hot under the collar, when drunk he'll say he's had one over the eight, when depressed he'll be described as having a face as long as a fiddle, and when feeling ill he may describe himself as feeling a little queer. All these expressions leave room for misunderstanding.

The problems of dealing with patients are naturally accentuated when they do not have the same national or cultural background as the doctor. There were in the town quite a number of immigrants from Europe. Apart from the Pirelli family, there were the Chlowski family from Poland, the Nagy family from Hungary, the Brauns and the Hubers from Germany, and the Adlers from Switzerland. Most of these people did, however, speak a little English. Those patients who came from Asia sometimes spoke almost none. Under such conditions medical practice takes on some of the aspects of veterinary practice.

When I first met Mr Singh I decided that he had some of the symptoms of Parkinson's disease. His face seemed blank and devoid of expression, his shoulders were hunched together, he shuffled along in the typical gait of the Parkinsonian patient, and his fingers had the almost pathognomonic tremor characteristic of the disease.

Since the tremor disappears when the patient attempts to use his hands I wanted to see Mr Singh do so. I sat down on the desk beside his chair and began to scribble an imaginary letter.

'Now you try,' I suggested, handing him the non-existent pen and pointing to the non-existent piece of paper.

He looked at me as if worried about my mental state.

'Which hands do you work with?' I asked him. I picked up an imaginary hammer and hammered an imaginary nail into my desk top.

The unhappy man stared at me dully.

'You try,' I suggested, pointing to him.

'No!' he begged, jumping up and moving away from the desk.

With some difficulty I persuaded him to sit down again. This time I decided to try a more social activity. I picked up an imaginary beer-glass and raised it to my lips. I then drained it noisily and wiped the imaginary froth from my mouth. I pointed to him again and raised a questioning eyebrow.

'Yes,' he nodded, staring at me without a smile. 'Yes, please.'

I decided to start him on L-dopa, relying simply on my diagnosis without prolonging the agony of clinical examination. I prescribed a month's supply of tablets and told him to return when it had been exhausted. He came back a week later, bringing with him a fellow-countryman.

'Where have all the tablets gone?' I asked, directing my question at the friend, whom I hoped would have some English.

Neither said anything.

'Do you speak any English?' I asked the friend.

'Interpreter,' he explained with a broad grin.

'Ask him where his pills are.'

'Please?' asked the interpreter, with an even broader grin.

'The pills,' I said. 'Where have they all gone?'

He turned to Mr Singh and spoke to him for several minutes. I waited for the outcome. Eventually he turned back to me.

'The pain is on the whole around the area of the arse,' he said unexpectedly. He pronounced the word 'arse' as if he had absolutely no idea at all that it might not be suitable for polite company.

'What has happened to the pills I prescribed?' I asked again.

Once more the interpreter turned to Mr Singh and once more he spoke to him for several minutes. Mr Singh grunted several times, but the conversation was unintelligible to me.

'Much pain in the twig and berries,' the interpreter said firmly. He turned back to Mr Singh, who nodded his solemn agreement.

'Take off your clothes,' I said to Mr Singh, hoping to discover the cause of his painful twig and berries.

The two men sat and stared at me.

'Take your clothes off,' I said, leaning forward and unfastening Mr Singh's tie. He understood and got up. He seemed confused but walked across the surgery to the couch. Congratulating myself on this minor victory I waited for him to disrobe. It was a lengthy business. When he'd finished I turned round to pick up my stethoscope. The interpreter had also taken his clothes off and was standing, totally naked, beside my desk.

'Not you,' I told him – rather brusquely, I'm afraid.

I examined Mr Singh carefully but could find no explanation for his pain.

'Please get dressed,' I told him, handing him his vest. Obediently he began to do so.

As I turned away from the examination couch I noticed that the interpreter was still standing there. It was not difficult to see that he had an enormous hernia stretching down into his scrotum.

'How long have you had that?' I asked, pointing at it.

'Five year,' he said, holding up a fistful of fingers.

'You understand?' I asked, quite surprised.

'Interpreter,' he explained, 'at police court.'

'Very good,' I congratulated him. 'Now I'll arrange a hospital appointment for you. You have an inguinal hernia. It isn't a major problem, but you need an operation to repair it.'

'Very good,' he agreed.

'What's your name?' I asked him.

'Patel,' he told me. 'Shall I dress?'

'Please do.'

'I appreciate you seeing me,' he said slowly, with a gracious nod of the head, as he was reclothing himself.

'It wasn't difficult,' I said ambiguously.

'My friend recommended me,' he explained, pulling on his trousers.

'What's he done with all his pills?' I asked yet again.

The two Indians began once more to talk together. The conversation lasted for several minutes, as seemed to be the case with all conversations in their tongue.

'Why do you ask this?' asked the interpreter.

'I gave him enough pills for one month,' I explained.

'Yes,' agreed Mr Patel. 'Mr Singh says that exactly.'

'So why did he come back today?' I asked. 'Has he finished all the pills already or is there some other problem?'

'There is no problem,' said Mr Patel. 'Mr Singh came with me as friend.' He put on his jacket, adjusted his shirt-collar and held out his hand.

We said goodbye.

After they had gone I sat and thought about the consultation. Mr Singh, it appeared, had brought Mr Patel along to the surgery because he had been pleased with the attention he had received. It was hardly surprising that Mr Singh had been surprised when I had insisted on his undressing for examination. I had learnt that when there are language problems you cannot even be sure which patient is the patient.

But within seconds of their leaving I realised I did not have Mr Patel's address. I had no idea where either of them lived. I chased after them and caught them up just outside the surgery.

'Where do you live?' I asked Mr Patel breathlessly.

'With him,' he said, pointing to Mr Singh.

'Where does he live?'

He started to stab his forefinger into his own chest but thought better of it.

'Why do you want that?' he asked suspiciously as he backed away from me.

'To get in touch with you,' I explained, 'about the hospital.'

'Oh no,' he said, beginning to run. Mr Singh ran with him. I chased after them for fifty yards or so but gave up when I realised I still had my carpet slippers on and that it was beginning to rain.

I quite forgot about the pair until, a week or so later, I had a visit from Sergeant Martin.

'Sorry to bother you, Doctor,' he apologised, 'but we're making enquiries about some Indian gentlemen.'

'Yes?' I said hesitantly.

'You see, there's been a good number of illegal immigrants in the town,' he explained. 'Have you seen anyone new in the area recently?'

Had I taken Mr Patel's address I might have been in something of an ethical quandary, but as it was I was able to tell them only that one of the men they sought had a little discomfort in the region of his twig and berries.

Sergeant Martin, whose command of English vernacular, it seemed, was worse than mine, looked up as he wrote down my statement.

'Could you spell twiganberries, please, Doctor? I'm not too hot on these medical terms.'

Mr Pirelli came back at the end of the week.

'Backamuchabetta,' he told me with a great beaming smile which showed off his excellent teeth.

'Splendid.'

'Resta O.K.' He nodded cheerfully.

'Good,' said I.

'I go to work,' he suggested.

The ability of a patient to resume work after a physically incapacitating illness depends, of course, upon a the physical demands of the job. A builder's labourer will need more rest after a backache than an accountant will.

'What is your job?' I enquired.

'I lika you,' said Mr Pirelli.

'That's very nice of you,' I said, blushing.

'Very much lika you!' he repeated. He was pleased with himself and slapped his thigh loudly.

'Very kind of you,' I murmured, rather embarrassed.

'I do like you do!' he guffawed, now roaring with laughter. He prodded the desk with a podgy forefinger and held his stomach as he laughed at his wit.

'What exactly is that?' I asked him.

'Withapatients,' he said. 'Buta my patients they no speak!'

Again he roared with laughter. I smiled at him tentatively. I wasn't so sure that my patients talked to me, either. 'You work with animals?' I enquired.

'Animals?' He lay across the desk and wiped tears from his eyes. 'Good that, animals.' He convulsed with laughter and his body jerked away from the desk. As it did so he gave out a great yelp. 'Aaaah!' he cried. 'Myabacka!' The tears of joy turned to tears of pain.

I laid him down on the couch and gave him two pain-killing tablets. Half an hour later as I helped him out of the surgery I asked him again what his job involved. He told me that he worked for a local firm of undertakers.

18

THE RUNNER BEANS had begun to flower, the peas were in pod, the lettuces had been eaten and the radishes were but plump succulent memories. Margaret and I were well pleased with our gardening; there is something intensely satisfying about being able to eat food one has grown oneself. The doctor's life, although rewarding in many ways, is never creative. The very best a doctor can hope for is to restore people to the health they enjoyed before. The general practitioner stands by the roadside as people trudge through life; it is his job to effect running repairs and, when possible, put the wounded and weary back on to the road. The magnificence and wonder of child-birth form a miracle which only very rarely owes much to medicine.

But turning tiny seeds into fully grown vegetables is, despite the inevitable support from God, a rewarding and pleasing occupation. There is, of course, a great deal of drudgery involved in looking after a garden of any size. Such tasks as weeding, mowing the lawn and clearing away leaves and dead flowers all take time and energy. On almost any weekend morning the sounds of water splashing on to the family saloon are almost drowned by the steady phut-phut of the motor mower and the irregular curses emanating from the gardener tending his roses. Roses never seem to understand that the hand which prunes and weeds is trying to be helpful.

The task I found most daunting, however, was the trimming of an enormous privet archway which stood in the centre of the garden and which had no appreciable practical function apart from acting as a shelter for a small white painted iron bench. I had put it off for several weeks, but eventually I could no longer ignore the fact that it was rapidly becoming bedraggled and untidy.

We had already purchased an electric hedge-trimmer and

an immense length of cord. 'It's better to have too much than too little,' Margaret had said as we struggled home with the reel. 'There's nothing worse than having a cord that's just a foot too short.'

I remembered her comments as I ripped open the cord's polythene package and allowed the contents to spill out on to the lawn. During the next few minutes I discovered just how malignant ordinary electric cable can be. As I carried the hedge-trimmer to the archway the cord managed to sew itself into an extraordinary creation which, if worn by a model in Paris, would have been decried as far too enveloping.

After ten minutes or so spent attempting to disentangle it I decided to get on with trimming the privet. Unfortunately I found that even when standing on the bench I could not reach the top of the archway. I put down the trimmer, went to the garage and found a handsaw. I then started cutting out some of the branches at ground level, thinking that perhaps that would prove a suitable and sensible alternative to tidying the top of it. Only when I had cut down thirty or forty thick stems did the stupidity of what I was doing become clearly apparent. The archway now consisted of a number of isolated stems which still reached far too high into the sky and which were just as untidy as they had been when I started.

I was sitting on the bench contemplating the huge pile of privet that I'd cut down and the huge tangle of cord when the telephone rang. Seconds later the doorbell, unwilling to be left out of things, rang too. Thankfully, I rushed indoors. Margaret had already started for the doorway, so I attended to the tele-phone.

The caller asked me to visit Mrs Phoebe Bridges. She knew nothing about Mrs Bridges' infirmity and could give me no information about the need for the visit. 'I'm Mrs Bridges' cleaner,' she explained. 'She just telephoned me and asked me to give you a ring.' She had no idea why Mrs Bridges should have called her and not rung me directly.

I was pulling on my coat and looking for the car keys when Margaret came into the kitchen. She brought with her two small boys in short trousers. They both wore Boy Scout uni-forms. 'These two young men want to know if we can give them any jobs to do,' she said. 'They're raising funds for a new clubhouse. I thought I'd let them do some weeding and tidying up in the garden.'

I kissed her, patted the two young gardeners on their heads, found the car keys in my trouser pocket, and set off. Mrs Bridges lived in a huge mansion of a house which must have kept her cleaner as busy as the painters of the Golden Gate Bridge. But at least it wasn't difficult to find.

There was a note pinned to the front door. I unpinned, unfolded and read it.

'WALK IN, DOCTOR,' it said, 'THE DOOR IS OPEN.'

When I pushed at the door it swung easily inwards. I stepped gingerly into the hall. I'm always slightly nervous about walking into other people's homes. You never know when a Dobermann pinscher is going to come leaping out from behind a chaise-longue, grandfather clock or escritoire.

Looking around I saw another note pinned to the bottom step of the staircase. I bent forward and picked it up. The visit was beginning to take on the air of a party game or treasure hunt.

'UPSTAIRS' was the bald message on this note. Like that pinned to the front door, it was written on scented notepaper in purple ink. I climbed the stairs. The landing looked like a display centre for doorways. There were no less than nine, and all of them were closed.

'Mrs Bridges?' I called tentatively. There was no reply. I looked at the two notes in my hand to reassure myself that I was at least in the right house. At the very least the occupant was clearly expecting a visit from a medical practitioner.

As I stood there various awful possibilities occurred to me. Perhaps Mrs Bridges had suffered a fatal heart attack and was now lying dead behind one of those nine doors. Perhaps she had called for help in a depressive state and was lying across some blood-stained mattress with both wrists slashed and the knife still moist. Perhaps, I thought, she had been murdered by some intruder.

The notes, which suggested a more leisurely onset of symptoms, were my only comfort. Eventually, plucking up all my courage, I began to open the doors. It was, almost inevitably, the seventh door that finally led me to Mrs Bridges. It led to the bathroom, where a woman was lying in a steamy bubbly bath with only her head visible.

'Do come in, Doctor,' she said. 'I'm glad you found me all right.'

I moved farther into the bathroom.

'Would you be kind enough to shut the door?' murmured Mrs Bridges. 'There's a terrible draught.'

I did so and put my black bag down on a small stool.

'What can I do for you?' I asked her. 'What's the trouble?'

'Would you like a drink?'

'No, thanks,' I said. 'I'm driving.'

'I'll have a gin,' she said. She lifted a hand from the bath and pointed to a small cupboard above her head. 'There's a bottle and a glass in there.'

I poured her a measure.

'I've got this most dreadful pain,' she said, sipping her gin with all the delicate caution of a thirsty man in a desert handed a glass of water.

'Whereabouts?' I asked her.

'Every time I go for a tinkle,' she said. She lowered her eyelids and studied her almost empty glass with unnecessary care. Although she would probably never see her fortieth birthday again, she looked embarrassed.

'You mean when you pass water?' I suggested, exchanging one euphemism for another.

She nodded.

'How long has this been going on?' I asked.

'Since last night.' She held her glass out to me. I filled it for her again, although it didn't seem a good idea if she had a bladder infection. I hadn't the courage to argue with her.

'Are you going out a lot?' I asked her.

'I went to a bit of a party last night.'

I moved my bag off the stool and sat down.

'Met this gorgeous fellow,' she went on. 'I think perhaps he was a little rough with me.'

'It's hot in here, isn't it?' I said, wiping my sweating brow with my handkerchief.

'You don't think I could have got anything nasty from him, do you?' she asked.

I muttered something about honeymoon cystitis. She giggled.

'Not exactly my honeymoon, darling.' She smiled. She winked, and an eyelash which managed the trip down didn't quite make the trip up. It slipped down into the bathwater and floated there like a drowning spider. I couldn't take my eyes off it.

'Just drink plenty,' I suggested. 'We'll have to see how it goes.' Mrs Bridges who'd emptied her glass again, handed it to me. I handed it back. 'But not too much alcohol,' I told her. 'It'll make the pain worse.'

'Spoilsport,' she said.

'I must be off,' I said, standing up.

'Oh, don't go,' she said. 'There's lots more I wanted to ask you.'

I sat down.

Suddenly, without warning, she sat up. The water-level dropped, leaving her chest covered in an uneven layer of bubbles which could not hide the fact that she was well enough endowed to keep a notebook hidden, let alone the proverbial pencil.

'I want you to have a look at my chest,' she said, wiping the bubbles away.

I looked at it.

'What do you think of it?' she asked.

'It looks fine,' I said. 'Was there anything in particular that worried you about it?'

'One of my boyfriends thinks my breasts are too big,' she said. 'What do you think?'

Before I could reply there was the sound of a door being slammed downstairs. Mrs Bridges leapt out of the bath and clamped two wet hands to my shoulders.

'Quick!' she said. 'That'll be my husband. You must go.'

I stood up totally confused.

'He's very jealous,' she said. 'If he catches you, he'll kill you.'

I began to protest, but the thought of Mr Bridges wielding a blunt instrument suggested to me that flight would be more sensible than explanation. The neurotic and septic Mrs Bridges would probably do little to help my honourable alibi. The general practitioner is always at risk when caught with someone else's pants down.

I left the house as if it were on fire and didn't stop trembling until I was a mile away. Then I sat in the car and waited for my heart rate to go below 150 again. Eventually, when it had slowed a little, I started off once more. Without my noticing it the sun had come out, and I drove home with the window open, enjoying being alive and out of prison. I never once looked at my speedometer and it wasn't until I arrived home that I realised that I had been followed by a police car.

'Think you're in a Grand Prix?' demanded a spotty youth in a police uniform swaggering round to my window.

'I'm sorry . . .,' I began.

'Bit late to be sorry,' said the policeman with a sniff. 'You were doing thirty-seven miles per hour back there in a restricted zone.' He sniffed again. 'Sir,' he added without much enthusiasm.

'I was coming. . . .'

'Yes, yes,' he interrupted. 'I've heard them all. This is your car, I take it?'

'Of course it's my car.'

'What's the registration number?'

'I don't know,' I confessed. 'You can't see it from inside the car.'

'Can I see your driving licence?'

'I'm sorry, I haven't got it on me,' I said. 'I'll go and. . . .'

'Oh, we *have* got a one here, haven't we?' said the policeman. 'Taking and driving away a motor vehicle. Driving without a licence. Get the book, you will.'

Just as I was beginning to see myself breaking stones in some deserted prison yard a second police car drew up. The arrival of the reinforcements did nothing to allay my fears until I saw that the driver was Sergeant Martin.

'Hello, Doctor,' he said kindly.

'Hello, Sergeant,' I replied. Now an open prison seemed much more likely.

'Exceeding the speed limit in a stolen car with no licence,' said the spotty young policeman.

'This is your car, isn't it, Doc?' said the sergeant.

I nodded.

'Visiting a patient?'

I nodded again.

'That's all right, Wormald,' said Sergeant Martin. 'This is

Doctor Vernon. You can buzz off now. The traffic lights at Ferry Road aren't working.'

Disappointed, the spotty policeman climbed back into his car and drove off.

'Thank you, Sergeant,' I said.

'Not at all,' he replied. 'Try to keep it down a bit will you, though?' he added with a wink.

'Right,' I agreed.

'I should wind your window up if you're leaving the car there,' he suggested. I did so.

Unfortunately neither he nor I had noticed that the end of my tie had been blown through the open car window. When I'd wound up the flap it had been tightly caught.

I slammed the door and very nearly strangled myself.

He helped me indoors and within a few minutes my colour had returned to normal. I was sitting in the kitchen with him and Margaret, drinking tea, when the two Boy Scouts appeared at the back door. They both looked very pleased with themselves.

'We've done the weeding,' said the first one.

'And we've picked you some flowers,' said the second. With a flourish he produced a small posy consisting entirely of the pretty red blooms from our runner bean plants.

The presence of the sergeant probably saved the boys' lives.

19

IF THIS WORLD WERE IDEAL, every male patient entering a doctor's surgery would wear a pair of swimming-trunks and every female patient a bikini. Such brief costumes would enable doctors to examine patients without the lengthy delays which take place when buttons have to be coaxed back through button-holes, zips tugged back across wastelands of escaping flesh and corsets wrestled into submission.

The laws of everyday medical practice are such that invariably the man with an ingrowing toe-nail will wear a pair of tightly fitting lace-up boots and the woman with piles will wear combinations, a corset and all the other protective impedimenta of the cold and figure-watching female. Women attending ante-natal clinics or coming for repeat prescriptions of the contraceptive pill, and needing to have their blood-pressure taken, usually wear dresses with tight-fitting sleeves. When the layers of clothing have been peeled away like the outer skins of an onion the ostensibly fat patient will often turn out to be dangerously thin.

Some patients, of course, undress without any problem and without appreciable delay.

Miss Sylvia Silhouette came into surgery complaining of a cough which had peristed for several weeks. 'It's most embarrassing, Doctor,' she said. 'In my job you just can't stop and have a cough when you need one. It spoils the atmosphere.'

'What's your job?' I asked innocently.

'I'm in show business,' she told me proudly.

I looked up. 'Very nice.' I smiled. 'I don't think I've ever treated a celebrity before.'

'Oh, I wouldn't say that I was a celebrity yet,' she said modestly. 'Most of my work is local, although I have had enquiries from farther afield.'

'Do you sing?' I asked.

She shook her head, and answered that regretfully her singing talents had not so far been appreciated or recognised to their proper extent.

'What sort of act do you have, then?' I asked her.

'It's a speciality act,' she said. 'You could say that my body is my fortune.'

'Ah,' I said. 'You, er. . . .'

'I'm a stripper,' said the patient, with unexpected honesty. 'I do the workingmen's club. Twice a night and three times on Sunday.'

'How long have you had the cough?' I asked – rather abruptly, I fear.

'Three weeks,' she answered. 'I've tried all sorts of things from the chemist's, so don't just give me a bottle of medicine, will you?'

'Have you been short of breath?' I asked.

She nodded. 'I am if I move about a lot. The stage isn't very big at the club, so it isn't too much of a problem there, but I play for the Church Volley Ball Ladies Team and I get awfully short of breath.'

'Any pains?' I asked her.

'A few,' she admitted.

'I'd better examine you,' said I. 'Do you mind taking your things off?'

'Don't see why not, luv,' she said. 'If you can get rid of this cough, you deserve a free show.' She unbuttoned her jumper and stood up, sliding her arms out of the sleeves with seductive ease. The dress she wore had clearly been designed for someone of more modest proportions. I took a sudden and unusual interest in a blank piece of blotting-paper as she undressed, terrified lest she ask for my assistance. Her movements were so easy and fluid that I waited expectantly for the music to start. She undid the last button and the dress dropped suddenly to the floor. Underneath she wore a pair of black stockings, a garter belt and a pair of briefs which were decorated with a large red silk rosette. From the waist upwards she was quite naked.

'They're not bad, are they?' she asked.

'No,' I answered automatically, realising as I spoke that my attention had been distracted from the blotting-paper despite the advertisement on the back of it which offered up-to-date information on the indubitable values of Unicorn Pedicure cream.

'Six hundred quid,' she said in hushed tones. She lifted three hundred pounds' worth up a couple of inches and then allowed it to fall back into place. It wobbled hardly at all.

'Marvellous,' I sighed.

'Still, I save on bras,' she said, admiring the other three hundred pounds' worth. 'You can't see the scars, can you?'

I admitted that the surgeon responsible had left virtually no signs of his activity.

'My boyfriend loves them,' she said. 'That reminds me,' she added. 'You're used to giving out advice. Can you help me?'

I sat patiently and awaited the next symptom.

'I've bought my boyfriend some new cufflinks. Would you tell me what you think of them?' she asked, leaning forward and picking up her handbag. 'The jeweller said I could take them back if I wasn't sure about them.' She opened the bag and took out a small red leather box. From inside that she took a pair of solid-gold cufflinks, each carrying a single large ruby.

I had to admit that I know little or nothing about jewellery and that the qualities of ruby-encrusted gold cufflinks are something I am not in a position to judge. I did, however, assure her that I thought the prospective recipient would be delighted with such a magnificent gift.

'Let me listen to your chest,' I begged, picking up my stethoscope and placing the ear-pieces in position. Miss Silhouette put the cufflinks down on the couch and stood up stiff as a ramrod. Her mechanically aided bosom stood out like the wooden mascot on an eighteen-century galleon. With considerable difficulty I managed to manœuvre the stethoscope around those well-balanced banks of breast.

'You need an antibiotic,' I told her eventually, standing back and turning to my desk. 'You can get dressed now.'

Her sudden squeal was so sharp that my first thought was that she had somehow suffered a puncture. Turning to face her, I found her pointing to the couch upon which lay a single cufflink.

'There's one missing!' she cried.

'Well, it must be around somewhere,' I assured her. 'It must have fallen off the couch.' We both bent down to look for it.

'There it is!' she said with relief. She pointed underneath the couch. We bent down together and reached for it. We were both half under the couch when someone knocked on the door.

'Come in,' I called automatically.

'There's a leak in the kitchen — Oh,' said Margaret, a sudden iciness creeping into her greeting. 'I'm sorry. I didn't realise you were so busy.'

'We were looking for Miss Silhouette's cufflink,' I explained limply.

'Of course,' said Margaret very sweetly. She smiled at Miss Silhouette and backed out of the surgery. 'Perhaps you'd pop out when you've found it.'

'How pretty,' said Miss Silhouette. 'Your secretary?'

'My wife,' I replied.

She giggled infuriatingly. As she dressed I wrote out her prescription.

'I'll come back if it doesn't get better,' she said. I wasn't sure whether it was a threat or a promise.

I found Margaret standing in the middle of the kitchen holding an old towel on to the ceiling with a broom-handle.

'There's a leak,' she said coldly.

'She really had dropped a cufflink,' I assured her.

'I think it's in the bathroom.'

'We were both looking for it.'

'I think you found it.'

'Don't be rotten. Honest, we were just looking for this wretched cufflink she insisted on showing me.'

'Honest?'

'Honest.'

'Did you like her. . .? Well, you know. . . . Did you like them?'

'I don't like artificial flowers, cream or breasts,' I assured her.

Suddenly Margaret let go of the broom-handle and threw her arms around me. We were both soaked as the sopping-wet towel fell from the ceiling followed by a gallon or two of warm water.

'It's warm!' I said. 'It must be the hot-water tank!' I rushed out of the kitchen and dashed upstairs. In the bathroom I found the bath full and overflowing. The bathroom floor was swimming with water, and the bathmat was floating towards the door. A half-floating loofa was jammed in the overflow pipe. Both taps were turned full on. I turned the taps off, pulled out the plug and went back downstairs.

'Were you going to have a bath?' I asked.

Margaret clasped her hand to her mouth in dismay.

'I forgot!' she cried. 'I came downstairs to find a fresh bar of soap and I got waylaid by one of your patients.'

As I set off on my rounds I decided to call in at the local book-shop and buy a new book on porcelain which I knew Margaret wanted. I parked the car outside the shop, walked across the road to the bank, cashed a cheque and entered the shop.

I found the book and handed it to the cashier with one of the brand new five-pound notes I'd collected from the bank. She examined the note as cashiers often do and checked its num-ber against a short list on a piece of paper taped to her till. It was something I'd seen happen dozens of times and I thought nothing of it until she called a colleague over and asked her to examine the note as well.

'It's a forgery,' announced the second girl.

'Let me see it, please,' I said.

'We can't do that,' said the cashier. 'We have to call the police.'

'But the note's still mine,' I pointed out. 'I haven't bought the book yet.'

'Sorry,' said the second girl. 'She's right. You'll have to wait until the police come.'

'But I've just got it from the bank.'

They were, however, insistent. Twenty minutes later the policeman arrived. He was a huge fellow accompanied for some reason or other by a minute policewoman. Both of them wore plain clothes, although the policeman had on his uniform trousers and shirt and his boots. Only his jacket belied his official role.

'Uttering a forged fiver, were you?' he said, poking his face into mine and breathing stale breath into my nose.

'I tried to spend that note,' I admitted. 'I got it from the bank a few minutes ago.'

The policeman laughed and took out his notebook. He

insisted on writing down my name and address and then record-
ing a lengthy statement in which I described where I had
obtained the note and what I'd intended to do with it. Eventually he let me go with a warning that I would be visited at
some future date and questioned further. I left without either
the book or the five-pound note and with very little dignity.

When I got back to the car a traffic warden was peering at
the number-plate and clearly just about to start writing me a
ticket. I ran across towards him hoping to point out why I had
been delayed.

'Oh, hullo, Doctor,' he said as I tapped him on the shoulder.
'I was coming to see you this evening.'

'Ah, very good,' I said, nodding idiotically. 'What can I do
for you? Save you a visit to the surgery.' I didn't recognise him
but was happy to take his word for it that he was a patient
of mine.

'I've got this cough my daughter's got,' he complained. 'You
saw her this morning and gave her some ampicillin.'

'This morning,' I said, still rather confused.

'Sylvia,' he said. 'Don't you remember her?'

'Oh, of course,' I said. 'You're Mr Silhouette.'

'Jones. Silhouette's her stage-name. Can I have some ampicillin?' he asked. 'I've got a shocking cough. Had it for weeks.'

'I'd better have a listen to your chest first,' I told him. 'Just
to make sure.'

'Here?'

'In the doorway there,' I suggested.

The traffic warden stepped back into a doorway behind him
and unfastened his uniform tunic. I poked my stethoscope
through the gap and listened for a moment or two.

'You've got a bit of a chest infection,' I told him. 'I'll give
you an antibiotic.' I took a prescription-pad out of the car.

Varying the treatment should, I reasoned, improve the
chances of getting a cure.

'Ampicillin?' asked the traffic warden.

'No,' I said. I didn't want him to think he could tell me what
to prescribe, and I didn't want him to think that my listening
to his chest had been a waste of time. 'I'll give you some tetra-
cycline,' I told him, knowing he would be unlikely to realise
how little there was to choose between the two drugs.

'Oh,' said he, impressed. 'Right.'

'Suit your cough better,' I lied.

He seemed duly pleased. I handed him the prescription as two pedestrians passed by, looking most surprised to see a motorist handing a traffic warden a piece of paper.

20

Outside Bulk Box Boards a dozen or more pickets were settled in deck-chairs, surrounded by radios, picnic hampers and hand-written paper placards and banners announcing that the firm would be 'blacked' as long as it continued to supply empty boxes to a firm supplying the régime in Guatemala with machine-tool parts.

Dr Williamson, who had been working as a general practioner in the town for two decades or more, was officially the company's medical officer, but his enforced absence on courses all round Europe meant that I, as his deputy for this purpose, received not infrequent invitations to visit the factory and treat the industrial wounded.

On most Monday mornings there would be half a dozen employees sitting in the canteen which served as the medical room and social hall. I quickly learnt that not all the employees took their work as seriously as their employer might have hoped. Dr Williamson would usually accept the suspicious stories put forward by men who were clearly itching to get off to a football match, but would occasionally satisfy his conscience by filling in their certificates with such phrases as 'plumbi oscillans' and 'haemodementia'; the former suggesting that the patient was swinging the lead and the latter that he was simply bloody-minded. These extraordinary certificates were apparently always accepted by the authorities, who never failed to pay out the expected funds.

I turned up one Monday morning, summoned to attend to the sick and weedy, to find the gates closed and guarded by a score or so of belligerent-looking young men I'd never seen before.

I stopped my car as three or four of them stood in front of me.

'Where ya goin'?' demanded one, poking his face through the window.

'Into the factory,' I answered. 'Why?'

'There's a dispute on,' answered a second picket.

'Well, I'm just the doctor,' I said. 'I'm not sure that my services are going to make any great difference to the success or failure of your cause.'

The pickets held a hurried roadside conference and eventually decided to let me through.

'Now, remember,' insisted one fiercely. 'There's no working on the machines allowed.'

I assured him as I drove past that I had no intention of operating any machinery other than my motor car and my sphygmomanometer.

Inside the canteen there was none of the usual Monday-morning bustle, and none of the usual Monday-morning coughing greeted my arrival. There was, however, a minute elderly lady who wore a pair of elegant pince-nez on her nose.

'You must be the doctor,' she said gracefully.

'I am.'

'My son is your patient.'

'Your son?'

'Mr Brand,' explained the old lady. 'I'm Lady Brand.'

I remembered that Mr Brand and his mother between them owned ninety-five per cent of the shares of the cardboard-box company. The news, which might otherwise have escaped my notice, had been announced in large red letters on one of the placards. 'I'm pleased to meet you,' I said, holding out my hand. Her ladyship, who clearly felt that shaking hands with the hired staff was a task considerably beneath her dignity, politely ignored my *faux pas* and turned on her heel.

'Follow me, Doctor,' she instructed.

Mr Brand's office came, as I had half-expected, out of a nine-teenth-century novel. The walls were covered with heavy pine panelling, as was the ceiling, and in the centre of each panel was an oil painting of one of the earlier Brands. The door itself was similarly covered and, once closed, was hard to find. The carpet was thick enough to deaden any sound, and Mr Brand's desk looked as though it had been carved out of a solid piece of oak at least large enough for conversion into an ocean-going raft.

'Good of you to come, Doctor,' he said, standing up as his mother showed me in. 'I thought that since we have little going on today I'd take advantage of the situation to have a bit of a medical.'

'But surely,' I began diffidently, 'your own physician. . . .'

'I haven't got a doctor,' he replied. 'Never have had. Can't stand them as a breed.' He smiled a little at that and offered me his hand. 'Nothing personal, you understand.'

'Quite,' I reassured him. 'Have you noticed anything wrong?' He was much thinner and older than I'd expected.

'Everything's wrong,' he cried vigorously. 'The trouble with this country,' he said, 'is that the spirit of adventure has been replaced by too much bloody milk of human kindness. What we need is more spirit and less damned milk.'

'Roderick!' said his mother sharply.

'Sorry, Mother,' he said. He turned to me. 'Mother's here helping me out while my staff are away on holiday.'

'On holiday?' I asked diffidently.

'The office staff,' he explained. 'I've sent them away on holiday for a week. Don't want them trying to get through that crowd of hoodlums every morning – and they would do.'

'What about the factory workers?' I asked.

'Oh, most of them are on holiday too. Those louts by the gates are all students. Most of my chaps bugger off to the seaside when we have one of these strikes. Gives me a chance to get the maintenance men in and have a bit of a tidy up. Surprising what you find. Last year we found twenty thousand pounds' worth of sheet cardboard stashed in the canteen. Found out later a chap had been selling the stuff to his mates for loft insulation.'

I must have looked disbelieving.

'We lost twelve wheelbarrows last year,' he protested vigorously. 'Found out a chap had been wheeling them out through the front gates as bold as brass. The chap on the gate looked in the barrow, saw it was empty and let him go through!'

'What I really want to know,' I pointed out, 'is whether there's anything wrong with you?'

Mr Brand said nothing.

'Any symptoms of anything?' I asked him.

'I've got lumps appearing all over my body,' said Mr Brand suddenly and unexpectedly. 'I don't know what it is, but there's something wrong with me.'

'How long have you noticed this?' I asked him.

'A couple of months.'

'Why didn't you tell someone before?'

'Never had much faith in doctors. Anyway, I've been too busy.'

'Have you noticed anything else?'

'I get tired very easily; I sweat a lot at night.'

'Let me examine you.'

'I don't want any of this medical bull about wonderful new treatments,' he said, taking off his jacket and glaring at me. 'Go and make some tea, Mother,' he said. When she'd gone he took off his shirt and tie. I examined him carefully. The enlarged lymph nodes were not difficult to find. There were some in his neck, more under his arms and others in his groins.

'I want to get some blood tests done,' I told him. 'And I'd like a specialist from the hospital to take a sample of one of those lumps and examine it.'

I telephoned from his office and arranged for a specialist at the hospital laboratory to look at some blood. I also arranged for a surgeon to take a biopsy of one of the lumps.

A few days later I had the results back. Mr Brand had Hodgkin's disease – a serious disorder of the lymph glands. I met him at the factory again and told him the news.

'I don't want to go into hospital,' he said. 'And I'm not having drugs pumped into me. I'm staying at home.'

I tried to persuade him to let me arrange for a course of deep X-ray treatment, but he refused adamantly. There was nothing I could do to make him change his mind.

'I want you to see me out when I can't get out of bed,' insisted Mr Brand.

'I can't do that,' I told him.

'You mean you won't.'

'I can't,' I insisted. 'But I will promise that you won't have any pain if it gets worse.'

'*When* it gets worse,' he said. 'I know what's happening.' He looked straight at me. 'It's not pain I'm frightened of. It's the indignities of death.'

I promised that he would suffer no indignities that were not necessary for his own comfort. After I'd left him I sat in my car as darkness grew around me. It was an hour before I drove away from the factory.

21

Mrs Young had been making good progress, and both the district nurse and I were well pleased with her. As I drove out to the village shop one Wednesday morning I considered the possible advantages of arranging for her to attend the local hospital's physiotherapy department. She still had difficulty in moving about easily, although her speech had returned and she was at least able to feed herself and see to her own basic needs.

When I got to the shop Mr Young was chattering enthusiastically to a tourist who'd strayed a little from the usual route. I was relieved to see that he was not confining himself to the sale of metal coathangers.

'It's a genuine nineteenth-century piece,' he insisted, fondling a rather battered chair with exaggerated care. 'Been in the family for years. Not for sale, of course.'

'Absolutely marvellous, don't you think, Elmer dear?' enthused a middle-aged lady in white trousers, dark-blue blouse and pink rinse. She wore, pinned to her blouse, a large cardboard badge which announced that she was Ida from Michigan and that she was touring with the Seymour Sights Travel Group, Inc.

'Used to be in the dining-room of William Shakespeare,' said Mr Young, positively caressing the chair. 'Probably sat on by the great man 'imself.'

'My oh my,' said Ida with a gasp of genuine astonishment.

'William Shakespeare!' sighed Elmer.

'Been in our family for generations, 'as this chair,' Mr Young told them. He saw me enter the shop and waved a faint greeting which seemed to suggest that he'd prefer me to postpone any interruption I might plan.

'May I sit in it?' asked Ida, with reverence in her voice.

'Well, you must go carefully,' insisted Mr Young. His caution seemed justifiable since Ida had a posterior of magnificent proportions which would have ensured her a considerable status in the African country where the beauty of a woman is measured by the size of her bottom.

Ida gently lowered herself on to the chair, which creaked its protest immediately. She jumped up straight away.

'My oh my,' she sighed. 'What a thing that is. I bet the Richardsons will be absolutely livid.'

'Shall I take a photo?' asked her husband, unwrapping a camera from around his neck.

As Ida gently lowered herself on to the chair again Elmer fiddled with his light meter and exposure calculator, and eventually pressed the button which would give the Richardsons permanent dyspepsia.

'Of course, I suppose I'll 'ave to sell it sometime,' said Mr Young with a look of convincing sadness. 'Times are very 'ard, you know.'

'Oh, we hear about your economic plight,' said Elmer, 'but we have our problems too, you know.' He seemed prepared to expound more fully the problems facing the American economy, but his wife was more concerned with helping Mr Young solve his immediate financial difficulty.

'How much would you sell it for?' she asked.

'Well,' sighed Mr Young, rubbing his chin thoughtfully and avoiding my glance with great skill. 'Well, now, that's a difficult one. I'd not thought of selling it at all.'

'How would we get it back?' asked Elmer.

'I can see you're attached to it,' said Mr Young quickly.

'Oh, it's lovely, Elmer,' insisted Ida, taking her husband's arm and smiling winningly at him.

'It is indeed,' he agreed.

'My wife would be very upset if she thought I was considering selling it,' Mr Young muttered, apparently to himself.

'Oh dear,' sighed Ida.

'But if I could buy her a new suite she'd soon get over it,' Mr Young added. He brightened up considerably. 'Yes,' he agreed with himself, 'if I could do that, she'd probably be 'appy enough.'

'How much would that be?' asked Elmer, taking out his wallet and producing a Diners Club card.

'What's that?' demanded Mr Young, peering at the proffered card with suspicion.

'A credit card.'

'Oh no,' said Mr Young. ' 'Aven't you any money?'

'Give him cash, darling,' said Ida. 'They don't have Diners cards here.'

Elmer took out a wallet of American Express cheques and a fountain pen.

'A 'undred,' said Mr Young.

'Dollars?' asked Elmer, pen poised.

'Pounds,' replied Mr Young, without flinching.

Elmer produced a small pocket calculator and converted the sum into dollars. He then wrote out traveller's cheques to settle the bill and handed them to Mr Young with a beaming smile.

'Here you are, sir,' he said. 'I hope you don't have too much difficulty persuading your wife that you've done the right thing.'

'I'll get round 'er, I'm sure,' Mr Young confirmed confidentially.

Elmer and Ida picked up the chair lovingly and carried it out of the shop. Mr Young didn't even offer to wrap it for them. I watched as the two customers struggled to pack it into the boot of their hired saloon car. They failed, and ended up tying down the boot lid with the belt from Elmer's safari jacket.

'I'm sure I saw some chairs like that outside the vicarage,' I said. 'The vicar didn't seem to think they were all that valuable.'

'That's the thing about the antique business,' he said without a flicker of a blush. 'It's difficult to tell the genuine article from the rubbish sometimes.'

Elmer and Ida waved cheerfully to Mr Young as they left. He waved equally cheerfully back.

'Well, how's Mrs Young?' I asked as he neatly folded his newly acquired traveller's cheques and pushed them into his hip pocket.

'She's not too good today,' he said with a shake of the head. 'She was doing fine until this morning. When I got up she seemed to 'ave slid back to where she was a week or two ago.'

'Oh dear,' I exclaimed with dismay. 'Let me have a look at her, then. Why didn't you say so before?'

'Well, I 'ad to make sure of that business deal, didn't I, Doctor?' said Mr Young. 'We all 'ave to earn an honest living.'

I followed him through the shop and into the cardboard-box-packed living-room where the smell of cabbage was as strong as ever. Then we went upstairs to see Mrs Young. This time I really wasn't happy about her at all.

'She's had another stroke,' I told Mr Young when all my attempts to contact his wife and to elicit signs of understanding had proved unsuccessful.

'What's caused that, then, Doctor?' he asked. 'I thought you said she was all right.'

'She was better,' I agreed, 'and I was very pleased with her, but I did say I couldn't guarantee that she wouldn't have any more strokes.' I paused. 'I think I'll have to send her into hospital. She needs specialist nursing care now.'

'Right,' he said. He sat down on the edge of her bed and to my great surprise burst into tears.

'We've been married twenty-five years,' he told me, pulling out an extraordinarily grubby handkerchief and dabbing fiercely at his eyes.

'She'll be better off in hospital,' I told him.

'I don't like 'ospitals, and neither does she,' he said. 'She's always been 'ealthy.' He put his handkerchief away and stood up. 'We're very close, you know, Doctor,' he said.

I said nothing but nodded to show that I was listening.

'We're neither of us much for showy affection,' he went on, reaching out and holding his wife's limp hand, 'but we do care, you know.'

I was touched and impressed by his obvious concern and sadness.

'If she needs any treatment you can't get for her ordinarily,' he said, looking very studiously at the bedspread, 'you tell me.' He swallowed hard and looked straight at me. 'I don't care how much it costs.'

Knowing what such an offer must have meant, I was even more impressed. 'I don't think you can buy anything for her that she can't get under the National Health Service,' I assured him. 'But if there *is* anything I'll tell you.'

I left him sitting beside his wife. She was breathing very slowly and had clearly had a sizeable stroke. I was not hopeful about her chances, but without hospital care she would clearly die. I drove straight back to the surgery and telephoned for an ambulance to pick her up. Then I realised that I hadn't arranged for the hospital to take her. I didn't even know whether or not they had a bed.

'Dr Barnes here,' said a rich, rather fruity young voice when I asked the switchboard operator to connect me with the house physician on duty.

'Dr Vernon,' I told him. 'Have you got a bed free for a female patient?'

'Ah,' he said. 'I'm not sure about that. Can you tell me something about her?'

'It's a lady in her late sixties,' I told him. 'She's the wife of a shopkeeper who keeps the village store in a little place just outside town.'

'Her clinical picture was what I really had in mind,' said Barnes rather haughtily.

'She's had a stroke,' I said baldly. 'Quite a bad one.'

'Where's the lesion?' he asked. 'Is it a thrombotic problem or a bleed?'

'Well, I'm not too sure, to be honest,' I confessed. 'But she's had a stroke.' I felt that I ought to be able to tell him more but, standing in Mrs Young's bedroom, a thorough neurological examination had seemed superfluous. I knew she needed to be in hospital. I told the houseman that.

'We don't usually take geriatric strokes,' he said. 'Too old. Not much we can do.'

'She's a lovely woman,' I told him. 'You could nurse her for a few days. She'll die if she stays at home.'

'Very tight bed situation,' he said. 'I'm afraid you'll really have to do the best you can at home. Can't you get the district nurse to call in?'

'I think this problem is too big for her.'

'Well, sorry, anyway.'

I was beginning to sweat. 'I'm afraid I've already got her in an ambulance,' I confessed. 'I didn't realise there would be a problem about getting her admitted.'

Dr Barnes said nothing at all. The silence was descriptive.

'She's on her way in,' I said. 'You'll have to turn the ambulance round and send her home.'

'I can't do that,' he snapped. 'What if she dies? There'll be all hell to pay. They'll say she died because I didn't take her in.'

'Well, if I leave her at home as you want me to, she'll die anyway.'

'Yes,' he agreed, 'but it won't be my responsibility.'

'So what do we do?'

'I suppose we'll have to keep her in,' he said with some reluctance.

I made a mental note to send all elderly patients requiring hospital care into hospital first and arrange for the hospital to accept them afterwards.

I'd just replaced the receiver when the surgery door burst open.

'I'm sorry, Doctor,' said Miss Williams.

'I want to see you,' said Miss Silhouette, pushing her out of the way and marching right up to my desk.

'I'm here,' I pointed out.

'I'm very sorry, Doctor,' repeated Miss Williams. 'She just walked in.'

'That's all right,' I assured her. 'I'll sort it out.'

'You'd better,' said Miss Silhouette. She glared at Miss Williams, who backed uneasily out of the surgery and gently pulled the door to.

'What's the problem?' I asked.

'You may well ask what's the problem!' said Miss Silhouette. 'I've just been laughed out of the Black Bull.'

'The Black Bull?'

'I was doing a special lunch-time show for a fellow's stag party,' she explained, kicking off her shoes. 'Look!' she shouted, unfastening her dress and pulling it up over her head in one swift movement. 'It must be your pills that have done this!' Her entirely naked body was covered in a fine red rash. 'It itches as well. I've never been so insulted in my whole career. I just pulled on my dress and came straight up here. It's those pills, isn't it?'

'Well, it could —'

'I knew it!' she yelled.

'It'll fade away quite quickly,' I assured her. 'You must be allergic to the antibiotic I gave you.'

'You'll be allergic to something!' she threatened.

'Stop taking the antibiotic,' I suggested, 'and I'll give you some antihistamine pills to stop the itching and help get rid of the rash.'

'I'm not taking any of your pills ever again!'

'But you'll need another antibiotic for your chest,' I protested.

'I'd rather have a bad chest inside than a bad chest outside,' she answered with considerable feeling. 'How would you like to stand naked in a pub with everyone laughing at you?'

I admitted that I would not find the experience enjoyable.

'I want a certificate from you to say the rash was your fault,' she insisted.

I wrote out a certificate confirming that it had been induced by pills I'd prescribed.

'And I want you to say that it isn't infectious,' she added. 'I've got a good reputation in this town.'

I added a postscript.

She took it out of my hand as I signed it, and headed for the door. She was halfway out into the hall before she remembered her dress. She dashed back into the surgery, picked it up and started to pull it over her head as she left.

Miss Williams poked her head in as the front door slammed.

'Are you in any sort of trouble, Doctor?' she asked quietly and solicitously.

'Miss Silhouette seems to think I've damaged her reputation,' I explained. 'I'm sure it will all die down in a day or two.'

'I hope it does, Doctor,' she said. 'I hope it does.' She shook her head and clucked. Dr Oaks had clearly never had such problems.

22

IT WAS SUNDAY, and Margaret and I were busy in the garden again. We'd started early, getting up at eight to try and regain control of the vegetable patch which, although designed and planted by human hands, had apparently been redesignated and replanted by more powerful forces.

Our first problem was to differentiate between the seedlings which we had put in ourselves and those which had insinuated themselves uninvited. At an early stage all plants look very much alike to inexperienced eyes. Then we were both astonished to see that apple-twigs which had been used as canes for beans and peas to climb up had themselves begun to sprout, and we carefully examined the wooden tongue-depressors, which we had used to mark rows of seeds, for signs of new growth. The cotton which we'd stretched across the peas to ward off marauding birds seemed to have acted simply as a guide rather than a deterrent. I stood and watched as a black-bird dived on to a patch of ground next to a couple of newly sprouting shoots, hopped over a piece of black cotton and pecked off the topmost and clearly tastiest parts of the plants.

'You can look after the vegetables,' I announced gloomily. 'I think I'll creosote the fence.'

'We need to dig over the scrub beside the compost heap,' Margaret reminded me. 'We were going to plant radishes there.'

'I'll ring the police and tell them I suspect that there's a human body hidden there,' I suggested. 'They might give it a good digging over for us.'

I fetched the creosote from the boot of the car and examined the label carefully. Margaret looked over my shoulder.

'It's dangerous,' I said.

'It says DO NOT SPLASH LIQUID ON TO SKIN,' she pointed out.

'And DANGER: KEEP AWAY FROM EYES.' I read. 'IF THIS

LIQUID IS SPILT OR SPLASHED INTO THE EYES SEEK MEDICAL AID
IMMEDIATELY.'

'Why?' asked Margaret. 'What would you do for it?'

'I haven't the faintest notion,' I confessed.

'In that case, you'd better stick to the peas and the radishes.'

'I'll wear sun-glasses,' I announced.

The telephone rang.

'Take your wellingtons off!' called Margaret as I rushed into the kitchen with unusual enthusiasm, leaving several great clumps of mud decorating the floor. I kicked off my wellington boots and padded in stockinged feet into the surgery.

'I'm trying to reach the doctor,' said a distant voice on the other end.

'Speaking.'

'Do you have a surgery today?'

'No,' I replied. 'Never on a Sunday.'

'I've got some spots.'

'How long have you had them?'

'Ever since they came out.'

'What day was that?' I sighed.

'Wednesday.'

'What sort of spots?'

'Well, I don't know – sort of spot spots.'

'Do they itch?'

'Yes.'

'Has anyone else you know got spots?'

'Yes.'

A caterpillar which I'd carried into the house on my jumper began walking slowly across the desk.

'What sort of spots have they had?'

'I don't know.'

'Have you got anything else wrong with you apart from the spots?'

'No.'

'Why didn't you get in touch before today?'

'I thought they might go away.'

'They still might.'

'I've got to go back to army camp tomorrow.'

'You're a soldier?'

'Private.'

The caterpillar began to climb up the side of my auriscope. I watched fascinated as it clambered slowly and carefully up what must have seemed to it like the Post Office Tower.

'I'm a private,' the voice said again. 'Are you still there?'

'I'm here,' I admitted. 'What do you want me to do about your spots?'

'If they're catching, I can't go back to camp,' he explained. 'It wouldn't be fair to take an infectious disease into the base. But if I don't go back I'll be posted Absent Without Leave.'

'So you need a letter from me?'

'I thought perhaps you might ring up my C.O.'

'You'd better come along to the surgery,' I said. The caterpillar had somehow climbed inside the auriscope and disappeared from view.

He thanked me and promised to come straight away. I put the phone down and hurried back outside to warn Margaret.

'I'll not be able to start anything too dirty,' I told her. 'I've got to keep my hands clean.'

'You can start creosoting your fence,' she pointed out. 'You've got to keep that off your hands, anyway.'

Intelligent women are all very well but they do have their drawbacks.

I was busily hunting for a brush when the doorbell rang. I abandoned the search and rushed back through the house to the front door. This time I remembered to kick my boots off outside the back door.

'Good morning,' I breezily greeted the caller. 'Come on in and let me have a look at them.'

'Pardon?' said the man on the doorstep.

'Let's have a look at them,' I said. 'Come on into the surgery.'

'Is there a surgery this morning?'

'Not a proper surgery,' I said. 'But I'll have a look at your spots for you.'

'I haven't got any spots.'

'You're not the soldier who telephoned a few moments ago?'

'No,' agreed the newcomer. 'I've been playing a football match in the Sunday-morning Summer League.'

'Oh.'

146

'I've cut my arm,' he said, holding out his arm and showing me a sizeable gash. Blood dripped from the wound on to the hall floor. 'Bad tackle,' he explained.

'It must have been.'

'I gave away a penalty,' he grinned ruefully.

'Did you drive here by yourself?'

'Yes. Everyone was too busy with the game.'

I led him to the surgery, sat him down and gave him a piece of gauze to hold on to the wound in an attempt to staunch the bleeding. I then rummaged around looking for some silk and needles to stitch it up with. Since Dr Oaks had left I had made several attempts to tidy and reorganise the surgery, but somehow my improvements rarely seemed to have any lasting effect. Within a day or two of every spring cleaning it was as disorganised as ever. I was beginning to suspect that it was simply doomed to remain as it had always been.

Eventually I found the silk sutures and the needles. The scissors, however, proved more elusive.

'Keep holding that firmly,' I said. 'I'll be back in a minute.' I went back into the hall, into the kitchen, and outside into the garden.

'You've forgotten to put your boots on,' said Margaret, pointing to my stockinged feet, which were planted firmly in a rather muddy patch of weeds.

'Have you seen the scissors?'

She thought for a moment. 'No,' she said finally. 'That reminds me. I couldn't find my kitchen scissors yesterday.'

'I need something to cut some stitches with.'

We both went back into the kitchen and began to search. At the door I took off my muddy socks.

'I've just remembered,' she said suddenly, with a beaming smile. 'I know where the scissors are.'

'Where?'

'I took them along to the ironmonger's to be sharpened. I've got to pick them up tomorrow.'

'All of them?'

'All of them. I was taking my kitchen scissors, so I thought I'd take yours as well.'

We hunted throughout the house and the only implements we could find which even vaguely resembled scissors were the garden edging shears. I picked them up and took them into the surgery.

'Sorry about the delay,' I apologised.

The footballer, still holding the piece of gauze on to his wound, stared at the shears and let out a horrified moan. He stood up and started to back towards the doorway.

'You're not taking it off?'

'These are for the stitches,' I said cheerfully. I explained the problem.

He thought for a moment, stared at the shears and then back at me, and gulped.

'Haven't you got anything else?'

'No.'

'A razor blade?' he suggested hopefully.

I was in the bathroom looking for a razor blade before I remembered that I shave with an electric razor. The journey was not fruitless, however. I found my nail scissors.

I stitched up the wound and gave him a tetanus injection. 'You'd better come back in five days and I'll take the stitches out,' I told him.

'Shall I come to you or go to my own doctor?'

'Aren't I your doctor?'

'Oh no, Dr Williamson's my doctor. But I didn't like to bother him since it's Sunday. Anyway, your surgery was nearer.'

I told him to go and see Dr Williamson towards the end of the week, and bade him goodbye. Then I went back outside to rejoin Margaret. I was hunting for the brush again when the doorbell rang a second time. I plodded back into the house, after kicking my boots off, and answered the door.

'Morning, sir,' said the caller. His smart but out-of-date blue suit and his short hair-cut clearly marked him out as a serving member of Her Majesty's Forces. He looked down at my bare feet and seemed slightly startled.

'Come in. Let me have a look at your spots,' I said once more.

He followed me into the surgery and stripped to the waist. He showed me a typical scabies rash.

'Is that bad?' he asked when I told him.

'No.'

'Can I go back to the base?'

'Not if they don't want infectious diseases,' I told him.

'Then it's good,' he said.

I took the number he gave me and telephoned his commanding officer.

'We don't want him here,' screamed the Commanding Officer.

I wrote out a prescription for some liquid, told the soldier to come and see me in a week and sent him on his way whistling cheerfully. The scabies mite is not, it seems, always an unwelcome visitor.

Sunday was beginning to seem more like Monday, and the garden looked just as unkempt as it had on Saturday. I restarted my hunt for a brush. This time I found one and was unscrewing the top on the large plastic bottle containing the dangerous stuff when the telephone went again. I removed my boots and padded back into the surgery. This time the caller was the sister on the women's surgical ward at the nearby district hospital. This, being far larger and more extravagantly equipped than the local hospital, was the place where more imaginative operations were usually performed.

'We have a patient of yours on the ward who'd like a word with you,' said the sister. 'A Mrs Young.'

'Mrs Young?'

'She says she's a patient of yours,' said the sister. 'You are Dr Vernon?'

'She is and I am,' I agreed, 'but she was in our local hospital.'

'They transferred her over here for major surgery,' she explained. 'She's having open heart surgery tomorrow.'

'Can you put her on?'

'I'm afraid not. This is our official line. Patients aren't allowed to use it. But you can come along to the hospital and see her.'

'Surely . . .,' I began. But arguing with hospital red tape is as unrewarding as arguing with any other type. 'I'll come over,' I said.

I put my boots on, went back into the garden, told Margaret where I was going, screwed the top back on to the creosote container, got into the car and set off for the district hospital. When I got there I parked the car in a space marked SENIOR CONSULTANTS ONLY and stuck my stethoscope around my neck.

A porter started towards me with a stern look on his face, but when he saw the stethoscope he faltered.

'Emergency,' I shouted, dashing past him.

Modern hospitals are stark, rather characterless places, in which it is very easy to get lost. The people who work in them always seem to be in a hurry and consequently visitors are usually reluctant to stop anyone for directions. Inevitably, therefore, the corridors are full of stray visitors and patients. It took me several minutes to find the women's surgical ward.

Once there, I introduced myself hesitantly to the neatly starched young sister in blue who sat in her office surrounded by files and flashing lights.

'Dr Vernon,' I said.

She did not reply, but stared in obvious astonishment at my feet. I looked down at my wellingtons.

'Gosh!' I said. 'You had me worried for a moment. I thought I'd forgotten to put my boots on!'

She still seemed to find some difficulty in saying anything. Eventually she managed it.

'You can't go into the ward in those,' she said, recovering her icy composure. 'Would you mind removing them?'

I took off the boots and padded on to the ward. Mrs Young was in a bed which, like the others, fitted snugly into a small private alcove.

'Hullo,' I smiled at her.

'Hullo, Doctor,' she said. 'Thank you for coming.'

'It's very smart here, isn't it?'

'I don't like it,' she answered.

'It's much smarter than our local hospital.'

'It's so lonely here,' she complained. 'I like to have someone to talk to. Something to see.'

'What are they going to do to you?' I asked, sitting down on the bed.

'Don't sit on the bed, Doctor,' she whispered. 'You'll get into trouble.'

I stood up.

'They want to operate on me. Should I let them?'

'What do they want to do?'

'I don't know,' she said. 'A doctor did try to explain, but I didn't understand.'

'You look a lot better than when I last saw you.'

'I am a lot better. My right arm and leg are a little weak, but that's all.'

I promised her that I'd find out what was planned for her, and went back to the sister's office.

'Can I see Mrs Young's notes?' I asked.

'I don't know about that,' said the sister coldly. 'That would be rather irregular.'

'I am her doctor,' I pointed out.

'Not here, you aren't,' countered the sister.

She was wrong, but I hadn't the courage to contradict her. Eventually she agreed to telephone the registrar and ask him to come and see me. He turned up ten minutes later looking very busy and professional in his crisp white coat. A bleep (as they're known in hospitals) stuck out of his top pocket, and his other pockets were stuffed with electronic and shiny chromium-plated gadgets. I explained again who I was and asked him to tell me about Mrs Young's planned operation. He looked at my grubby jumper, corduroy gardening-trousers and bare feet with undisguised revulsion.

'We plan open heart surgery for her,' he told me. 'She's got narrowing of her coronary arteries. She'll have a heart attack if we don't operate.'

'She's had two strokes,' I told him.

'She'll probably die otherwise,' said the Registrar.

'She's not certain whether or not she wants to have any operation, and she may die of a stroke even if you do operate on her heart.'

'I would have hoped that you would be on our side,' he said icily.

I told him that I wasn't on anyone's side; but I felt quite certain that, if I were, it wasn't his. If ever I'd been unsure about choosing a career in general practice as opposed to hospital medicine, I was now firmly convinced that I had made the right decision.

'What do they say?' asked Mrs Young when I returned to her bedside. I explained the problem.

'What do I do?' she asked.

'You must decide,' I told her.

'Advise me, Doctor,' she begged.

I felt confused and bewildered. On the one hand I felt that she would benefit little from heart surgery. With luck and good management she could probably live comfortably if somewhat restrictedly for several years. Would the operation help her live a more complete life? And was the risk worthwhile? And yet, on the other hand, I was fresh enough from hospital to be slightly awed by the Registrar, whose obvious expertise and technical knowledge were impressive. I felt that I owed him respect and professional loyalty.

I told Mrs Young that I felt she ought to have the operation. Then I held her hand and kissed her cheek. She clung to me tightly for a few moments.

When I got back, Margaret was sitting in the kitchen busily depilating an enormous basket of gooseberries. A man in a hairy tweed suit stood beside her drinking a cup of coffee.

'This is Mr Compton,' said Margaret introducing us. 'He brought us some gooseberries.'

'That's very kind.' I smiled.

'Patient of yours, Doctor,' said Mr Compton. 'Thought perhaps you'd have a look at my elbow for me.' He put his coffee-cup down.

'Ah,' I said. The gooseberries had to have a price. Still, they looked nice.

'Bit red and aches a devil of a lot,' he explained, taking off his jacket and shirt.

'Perhaps you'd like to come into the surgery?' I suggested diplomatically.

'That's O.K.,' he replied.

'I'm sure you'd be more comfortable there.'

'No, fine here,' he insisted.

To avoid further delay I examined his elbow there and then. It was indeed red, and slightly swollen.

'You've got a tennis elbow,' I told him. 'You'll have to rest it.'

'I don't play tennis,' he told me.

'Well, what have you been doing to get that arm?' I asked.

'I've done a lot of hoeing lately,' he explained.

'Then you've got a hoeing elbow,' I said. 'Rest it and come and see me in a few days if it doesn't get any better.'

He left. I gave him a small packet of anti-inflammatory pills to help relieve the pain and swelling.

Back in the kitchen Margaret was still struggling with the gooseberries.

'Can I borrow your electric razor?' she asked. 'These eyebrow tweezers are making my fingers sore.'

I couldn't think of a suitable reply. 'I'm going out to water the garden,' I told her, heading for the back door, 'before it starts raining.'

23

Mr Neville was the first patient to appear in the surgery next morning. He came accompanied by his six-year-old son Oliver. Mr Neville I knew well by now. Every time he came he unfolded complaints like a gourmet taking apart an artichoke.

'Oliver's swallowed a marble,' he said, pushing his young son forward.

'How big was it?' I asked Oliver, who seemed quite unaffected by his unusual diet.

'This big,' said Oliver, holding forefinger and thumb half an inch apart.

'You're sure it wasn't a great big one?' I asked him. To my horror I noticed that a caterpillar was slowly creeping out of my auriscope.

Oliver shook his head.

'That's no problem,' I told Mr Neville. 'It'll come through without any difficulty.' The caterpillar moved out a little farther. I quickly picked up the auriscope and put it in a drawer before Mr Neville noticed.

'But how do we get it back?' he asked. 'How do we know for certain that it's come through?'

'You'll have to keep an eye out for it,' I said. 'And then how you recover it is rather up to you!'

'H'm,' he said, clearly unhappy. 'Is that the best you can do, Doctor?'

'I'm afraid so.'

'How about an X-ray?'

I pointed out that the marble would probably not show up on an X-ray, anyway.

To my surprise, Mr Neville produced no other complaints. He stood up, took Oliver's hand and walked to the surgery door.

'Goodbye,' I called.

'H'm,' said Mr Neville. Oliver merely sniffed.

I spent the afternoon with Mrs Young at the hospital. She had had her operation and was lying in the intensive-care unit when I arrived.

'I'm so glad to see you, Doctor,' she said, grasping my hand and clutching it tight.

'How are you?'

'They say I've done very well. But, to be honest, Doctor, I'm frightened in here.' She looked around at the array of machines, television screens and highly coloured wires which festooned the room like electronic Christmas decorations.

'You'll soon be out,' I told her, and immediately regretted my false air of assurance. I had no idea whether or not she would soon be out of intensive care. 'I'll go and have a word with your doctor,' I promised her, 'and then I'll come back and tell you what he says.'

'Will you? You're not like a doctor,' she said. 'It would be nice to have you tell me what's going to happen.' I took the comment as a compliment and squeezed her hand.

The registrar in charge of the intensive-care unit was full of frightening jargon, as many doctors are these days.

'She's got a normal P.C.V. and C.V.P.', he said, 'but we're worried about her V.P.C.'s.'

'How is she?' I asked. 'Will she be able to go home soon?'

'That depends on her S.T. segments,' he replied. 'We're doing monitoring, and they're still raised, but we're cheerful. Her L.D.H. seems static.'

'Is she making a good recovery?' I asked.

'We're delighted with her S.G.O.T., and her E.S.R. is well within acceptable limits.'

'Has she got out of bed?' I asked. 'Is she eating normally?'

But apparently my questions were too complex. The answers revealed much about Mrs Young's physiological state but little about her clinical condition. Eventually I returned to her very little wiser.

'What do they say, Doctor?' she asked.

I sat on the bed and, in doing so, must have pulled a lead out of one of the machines which surrounded her. A television screen which had been showing a wave-like pattern suddenly showed a flat line and emitted a high-pitched squeal. A red light flashed on and off. Within a minute the room was full of doctors and nurses.

'Paddles!' ordered the registrar to whom I had been talking a few moments before.

'Lignocaine.'

'Sodium bicarbonate.'

'Drip set.'

The orders came thick and fast.

'She's breathing!' called a nurse, peering into Mrs Young's face.

'I've got a pulse!' cried a young doctor in a white coat and flowered shirt.

'I'm very sorry,' I said. 'I rather think this was all my fault.'

'You must have got her too excited,' said an officious-looking woman in a blue dress festooned in badges.

'Oh deary me,' and Mrs Young. 'I feel all faint.'

The team of life-savers seemed determined to do something to justify their existence, and I rather feared for her. I hunted around frantically among the bedclothes and eventually discovered the wire I'd pulled out. I found the jack-plug on the end of it and pushed it back into the monitor's only available socket. The screen immediately started to show a healthy wave-pattern again.

'She's off again!' I shouted, pointing to it.

'Sinus rhythm!' agreed a white-coated saviour gleefully.

The rest of the team stopped what they were doing and watched the monitor for a moment or two. Then they began to pack up their equipment. They looked like men and women well pleased with their expertise.

'Sorry about that,' I whispered to Mrs Young when they'd gone.

'I don't like it here,' she said with a shake of her head.

I told her to keep as quiet and patient as she could so that the doctors and nurses would get bored with her and send her home quickly. She agreed that that seemed the best solution, and gave me a big hug before I left. She asked me to give her a hug, too, so I took my chances with the General Medical Council and gave her a great squeeze.

I returned to the surgery to find that Margaret had a message for me from Mr Neville, asking me to ring him at home.

'What's the trouble now?' I asked.

'It's Oliver,' he said. 'His marble's come through.'

'Thanks for telling me,' I said, without much genuine appreciation.

'It cracked the lavatory pan,' he said.

I didn't say anything. There didn't seem to be much to say.

'You should have warned us,' he went on.

I still didn't say anything.

'You'll be hearing more about this,' he finished. He put the phone down and left me with a buzzing in my ears and a funny feeling in my stomach. I'd never been threatened by a patient before.

24

AFTER PORING OVER bundles of brochures with all the dedicated determination of someone preparing for a higher examination Margaret announced that we were going to Venice for our holiday. I protested mildly for a few minutes, pointing out that we couldn't really afford a holiday anywhere, let alone in Venice, but my protestations were shallow and short-lived – partly because I could see that Margaret had made her mind up and partly because I quite fancied going to Venice.

As a general practitioner with my own list of dependent patients, I did, however, have one important problem to solve before we could seriously contemplate a holiday. I had to find another doctor to take over the responsibility of looking after them. Dr Oaks had always managed to make arrangements with one or other of the local doctors who would provide emergency cover for a few days at a time. But because of their own commitments they had never felt able to do this for longer, and in consequence until my arrival Dr Oaks had not had a holiday of more than three days for many years.

Clearly Margaret and I would have to find a locum – a doctor prepared to come and take over the practice for ten days.

Now, doctors who do locums for general practitioners usually fall into one of two categories. They are either professional drifters, taking locum appointments at dozens of different surgeries during the year, or they are young hospital doctors seeking a little experience and more than a little money while preparing for higher examinations in some speciality.

Doctors in the first category are becoming rarer, but it is not their scarcity which is the problem so much as their inevitably unusual lifestyle. A doctor who prefers the roving life to the more usual settled existence of an established practice frequently has some private skeleton hanging in his cupboard, ready to leap out and startle everyone if the door is unfastened.

Doctors in the second category are more difficult to get hold of and produce problems of their own. Many an experienced general practitioner has gone away on holiday happily leaving his practice in the apparently capable hands of a bright young neurosurgeon or dermatologist and come back to find it in confusion and disarray. The technically astute young hospital doctor may find it disturbing to see hundreds of people regularly swallowing tranquillisers and vitamin pills for no apparent reason.

'You don't need those,' he'll insist sternly.

'But Dr McTiddle has been giving me them for twenty years,' old Mrs Ingram will insist. 'They keep me quite comfortable.'

The doctor will, however, remain adamant and Mrs Ingram will leave the surgery without her pills, wondering whether to believe Dr McTiddle or his locum.

I decided, however, that a doctor in the second category would be the safest bet and so I started to look around for a suitable candidate. I telephoned the local hospital first of all but no one there had any holiday which they were prepared to sell me. I then got in touch with the medical school where I'd been trained and asked the dean to put a notice up inviting any interested members of the hospital staff to telephone me.

To my surprise the advertisement brought an almost immediate response. I received a telephone call from a registrar at one of the hospitals in the teaching-hospital group.

'I hear you're looking for a locum,' he said when he'd introduced himself.

I confirmed that I was.

'It would suit me very well,' Dr Lewis assured me.

'Splendid,' I said. 'Can you come over so that we can meet?'

He agreed, and arrived an hour and a half later riding a huge and powerful motorcycle. He had a vast halo of curly hair and a pair of bushy sidewhiskers which seemed anxious to meet underneath his chin.

'I'm taking examinations in a few weeks,' he explained, 'and I've got one or two research papers I want to get written, so a nice quiet job in general practice will suit me fine for a while.'

'I'm not sure that you'll find the work quiet,' I told him. I didn't want to put him off, but I didn't want him taking the job in the mistaken belief that it would give him unlimited free time.

'It'll be a change to have patients who look straight at me,' he said, settling comfortably in the easy chair in one corner of the surgery.

I looked at him with a raised eyebrow.

'I'm a venereologist,' he said in explanation.

'Ah,' I said.

'I've got a month's leave due,' he went on. 'Bit of holiday and a bit of study leave.'

I told him when I hoped to be away. It seemed to fit in very well with the dates he gave me.

'Have you got a registration certificate?' I asked.

He looked at me a little puzzled.

'Not that I'm suggesting there's any doubt about your own qualifications,' I added hastily, 'but just for my own peace of mind. . . .'

'I'll post you a photocopy,' said the venereologist. 'And details of my Medical Defence Society membership.' He seemed rather offended but calmed down a little when I'd explained that I'd read of at least two practices which had hired car salesmen to look after their patients and been left with enough legal problems to keep a whole chamber of lawyers occupied for a year.

We shook hands. I tried to explain how the practice was organised and introduced him to Miss Williams. He roared off on his motorcycle.

'What on earth are you doing?' I asked Margaret when I arrived home from my evening visits one day shortly afterwards to find the hall littered wth bags and baskets.

'Packing,' she said.

'Packing?' I exclaimed. 'I thought you were spring cleaning.'

'Someone's got to get things ready,' she replied crossly.

'But we're only going on holiday, not emigrating,' I argued. I sat down on the edge of the umbrella-stand, the only piece of furniture I could see that wasn't already loaded with packets and boxes of clothes and miscellaneous holiday paraphernalia.

'How much of this stuff are we taking?' I demanded, picking up a large cardboard box which seemed full of books.

'All of it,' said Margaret, with suprise.

'We're only going for ten days,' I told her.

'It's all necessary,' she insisted.

I opened a carrier-bag and peered inside. It was full to the brim with packets of pills and capsules, bottles of medicine, tubes of cream and ointment, and jars of paste. There were several plastic syringes, numerous needles and a good variety of medical instruments. I closed it quickly and opened a brightly coloured plastic bag which advertised a major chain store. This, too, was full of medical equipment. A third carrier-bag contained an old microscope I didn't even know that I possessed. I looked round for Margaret and eventually spotted her kneeling down beside a huge cabin-trunk.

'We're flying, you know,' I told her. 'There will be other people on the plane.'

'It's all essential,' Margaret insisted again. She held up my sphygmomanometer. 'Do you think we need this?'

'I wish you wouldn't move things out of the surgery,' I told her. 'All my equipment seems to be wrapped up in paper bags.'

'We've got to take these things,' she said. She pointed out that, if either of us fell ill, we would need medical attention and that it would be silly to have to pay a foreigner high fees when I could, if properly equipped, do the job myself.

'Besides,' she said, 'there may be people ill on the aeroplane or in the hotel. It's only fair to be properly equipped if you're going to help them.'

I stepped over a large tin box which seemed full of drug bottles and knelt down beside her.

'We're going on holiday,' I reminded her. 'I have no intention of doing a morning surgery in the hotel lobby every day.'

'But emergencies,' she protested. 'What about emergencies.'

'Emergencies can happen anywhere,' I said. 'You're surely not suggesting that every time we go for a walk outside the hotel I carry all this lot with me.'

'Oh,' she said rather sadly.

'So let's put it all away.'

'What *shall* we take?'

'I'll pack the medical supplies.'

'Promise?'

'Promise.'

She began to unpack one of the boxes.

'What will you take?' she asked.

'Some aspirin tablets and a roll of sticking plaster.'

Our flight was due to take off at three in the morning and the holiday started with a slight problem. Margaret had packed her contraceptive pills in the suitcase which we'd handed in when we arrived at the airport. Then, as always happens when I travel by air, there was a delay. An aeroplane at Athens airport had lost a windscreen-wiper and consequently another aeroplane in Brussels had been diverted to Gibraltar with the result that ours had to be sent to Madrid to pick up a flight from South America that had been diverted to cope with a dozen stranded passengers in Dublin.

'I haven't taken my pill,' whispered Margaret anxiously as I dozed in the airport lounge, waking every five minutes to listen to the frenetic announcements over the loudspeaker system.

'What?' I muttered.

'Haven't taken my pill. I forgot, in all the excitement.'

'It's not evening yet,' I told her. 'Stop worrying.' I looked at my watch. 'It's only half-past four in the morning.'

'It's last night's pill I haven't taken,' said Margaret, shaking me awake.

I sat up.

'I put it in the suitcase,' she said sadly.

'And the suitcase has gone.'

'We can get it back,' she whispered.

Sighing, I stood up and struggled across the airport lounge to the information desk. The girl on duty looked bored and rather uninterested.

'You'll have to see the baggage desk,' she said. She added a 'sir' to the end of her sentence without much enthusiasm.

Airline employees always seem to me to be slightly put out when brought face to face with passengers. The staff seem determined to pretend they are just filling in time in between a modelling assignment in Paris and a film part in Hollywood. The porters never port and the stewardesses simply seem to be bad-tempered waitresses and saleswomen.

The man at the baggage desk listened to my sad tale without

any sympathy. 'Silly,' he said with a shake of his head. 'Very silly.'

'Can we retrieve the pills?' I asked him.

'Oh dear me, no,' he said with another, more vigorous shake.

'But we need them,' I pointed out. 'We need them now.'

'Should have thought of that, sir,' he said smugly.

'We didn't know your aeroplane was going to be delayed,' I pointed out.

'Contraceptive pills, I suppose?' asked the man with a leer.

'Who said they were contraceptive pills?' I asked him. 'This is a matter of life or death.' I felt Margaret pulling at my sleeve but ignored her studiously.

The man at the baggage desk looked a little more interested. I took my passport out of my jacket pocket and pointed to the line that said, 'Doctor.'

'These are important pills,' I insisted. 'Are you prepared to have someone die in your airport lounge because you refused to allow me access to our luggage?'

He blustered for a while, but he was defeated and he knew it. He disappeared with the stub of our baggage ticket and re-appeared half an hour later with a scowl and the case. I opened it, Margaret found her pills and I handed it back to the man with a smile.

'You said it was a matter of life or death,' said Margaret. 'That isn't true, is it?' She looked worried.

'Not because you've missed your pill,' I admitted.

'That was naughty,' she said. 'Telling a fib like that.'

'It wasn't a fib,' I told her. 'If we hadn't got those pills, that man might have died.'

She looked shocked.

'I'd have murdered him!' I grinned.

We finally arrived in Venice at midday. From the airport we rode in a water-taxi, arriving at our hotel half an hour later.

Venice must be just about the only major city in the world more or less unchanged by the invention of the internal com-bustion engine. It stands, like an elegant lady of position and breeding paddling at the seaside, outwardly unconcerned by the fact that the water, a little too high for comfort, is lapping about her skirts.

Every child knows that the streets of Venice are waterways, but it is only on arriving there that one finally realises just what that means in terms of peace and quiet. The absence of traffic noise makes Venice an ideal place for a relaxing holiday.

Margaret and I had booked into a hotel a few yards along the waterfront from St Mark's Square. From our bedroom window we could look out across the lagoon, kept remarkably busy with an unending stream of water-traffic. Merely abandoning our luggage, we wasted little time before setting off to explore. The whole island is criss-crossed with alleys and lanes so narrow that there can be barely room for an open umbrella in wet weather. Sometimes they stop abruptly at the end of a canal, sometimes at the back door to some great palace. The front doors are all approached by water.

We had been a little worried about the smell reputed to hang about Venice these days. We need not have been. Walking about the island was a continual delight, for so many tiny shops and factories are crammed on to the land that the smells of printers' ink, ground coffee, soap, candle wax, leather, roasting chestnuts and vanilla essence are all mixed up in one huge olfactory cocktail. I sometimes think that, rather than photographs or tape-recordings of the usual tourist sights and sounds, it would be fun to bring back smells. All cities have unique scents. In Paris it is the smell of the Métro; in fishing ports it is the smell of the early-morning catch, which lingers all day long; in the Black Forest it is the smell of the new-mown grass and the flowers littering the countryside; in London it is, I'm afraid, the far less romantic smell of rubber, oil and petrol mixed together. The odour of newly baked bread and the smell of an overheated internal combustion engine can bring back memories just as vividly as the sight of a member of the family.

There is much to see in Venice and the days never seemed long enough : the gondoliers with their strangely shaped craft cruising up and down the canals; the boatyard where the gondolas are made and mended; the hundreds of tiny shops stuffed to the ceiling with delicate, highly coloured glass ornaments, some of them beautiful, many quite excruciatingly hideous; the civil hospital where patients are brought in for treatment by boat and which, with a greater sense of practical need than of diplomacy, the Venetians have surrounded with funeral directors' establishments and printers' shops specialising in bereavement notices.

For both of us the cafés provided something special. In St Mark's Square, Florian's stands above its neighbours as a stylish and sophisticated centre for those who like to drink their coffee in good company – although, across the Square, Lavena is worth a visit. We spent many contented hours in both of these places, sipping our coffee and watching the wealthy Germans munching cakes and pastries we could not afford. (There was a time when the Americans were the financial aristocrats of Europe. Today it is the Germans.)

We sat there and talked about our first few months in general practice; our first few months of married life. A holiday away from the pressure of daily life is a wonderful opportunity to redefine hopes and ambitions. After the almost permanent state of siege at the surgery it was an opportunity to put things in order again, to prepare for the next six months' siege.

During those first months I had learnt a great deal about general practice. I had learnt that a general practitioner needs, above all else, common sense, which is nothing more than a combination of innate wisdom and experience acquired without any contaminating prejudice. I had learnt that the improbable in general practice is merely the extent of someone else's imagination. Nothing is impossible. I had learnt that general practice is jungle medicine as opposed to hospital medicine, which is zoo medicine, and that the two are vastly different.

I had learnt that patients like their doctor to have some air of mystery about him. For that reason I always wrote prescriptions with an illegible flourish, using a fountain pen and dog Latin abbreviations to dignify even the simplest. At the end of each consultation I would fold the prescription in two to give the whole process an extra touch of secrecy.

Dr Oaks told me once how he used to cultivate the feeling among his patients that he was slightly superhuman with the aid of a simple trick he described as sleight of mind.

'I used to forecast the sex of a woman's baby,' he told me proudly and with a wink, 'and never got it wrong.'

Fascinated, I asked him how he did it.

'I'd get the husband and wife together,' he explained, 'and I'd tell them their child was going to be a girl. Then I'd write down in my diary their name and the fact that their child would be a boy. I would let them see me writing, but I wouldn't let them see *what* I was writing. When the baby appeared, if it was a girl, they'd remember that I was right. If it was a boy, I'd produce my diary and show them the entry, insisting that they must have misheard.'

The old-style general practitioner had little in the way of powerful medicines and yet he did a great deal of good. Patients believed in his word. They respected him and did what he told them to do. The general practitioner today has more powerful drugs but less respect. The patients know their own minds and are more likely to reject or refuse his advice.

General practice was not entirely what I had hoped. But still I found myself beginning to think of my patients as members of some large family. There were parts of it I found confusing and annoying, but by and large I loved the responsibility for looking after it.

'If you weren't married to me,' I said to Margaret as we sat in Florian's one evening, 'would you marry me?'

'I'd marry you,' she said. 'Would you ask me?'

'I'd ask you,' I whispered.

The advantage of poorly lit cafés which are divided into many nooks and crannies is that honeymoon couples can canoodle a little without attracting an audience.

25

WHILE IN VENICE I grew a moustache. I had the idea while shaving on our first morning in Italy. I'd just finished clearing off the field of stubble which grows on my left cheek when it struck me that a moustache might look rather nice. Growing one at home might attract some comment, but on holiday who would care?

Once having decided to cultivate one, I had to decide on what type it should be. A small carefully cropped affair or one of those bushy creations favoured by airmen and comedians? Or perhaps one of those once fashionable moustaches which droop down on each side of the mouth and give the owner a rather doleful but serious look? I decided to grow a droopy moustache.

By the second day there was nothing at all to show for all the mental effort I'd put into it. I peeped into all the available mirrors and shop windows to study the rate of growth, and the only thing I could see was a publicity-seeking red pimple which had impertinently invaded the pitch.

By the third day I was convinced that I'd been shaving away for years quite unnecessarily. It was with some relief that I heard Margaret complain that evening, 'Haven't you shaved today?' I looked in the mirror and noticed a small grey shadow developing underneath my nose.

On the fifth day I decided to shave it off, although Margaret had guessed what was happening; for she, too, had started examining each day's growth with great interest. I actually got as far as lathering the site before my nerve failed me. I just couldn't destroy all that hard work. I wiped off the soap and turned away from the mirror quickly.

Slowly the thing took on a personality of its own. It became apparent from a distance of several feet that there was something there, that the something was too big to be an oversight, and that there was too much symmetry about it for it to be a complete accident. And then, on the day before we were due to travel home, I woke up with a moustache.

Miss Williams was the first person who ought to have noticed it. I walked into surgery early on Monday morning when we arrived back and waited for her to make some comment.

'Nice to see you back, Doctor,' she said. 'Did you have a good holiday?'

'Wonderful, thank you.'

'The locum managed quite well,' she assured me. 'But it's very nice to have you back again.'

'No crises?' I asked.

She shook her head. 'Nothing too bad. Miss Armitage fell over her poodle and broke her leg; Major Barwick got pleurisy and is in hospital; Mr Willoughby fell off his bicycle and grazed his leg; Miss George had her appendix out; and Mrs Trump had her fifth.'

'Nothing much different, then, really,' I said, stroking my moustache.

'Not a lot,' she agreed.

I pulled at the edge of my moustache.

'I'll be getting on, then,' she said, picking up a sheaf of papers and heading back towards the waiting-room.

The first major problem I came across was in the medical records, where our attentive academic locum had written careful voluminous notes on all the patients he saw. His handwriting was neat and easily readable, but I still couldn't understand his comments. It was the words he used. Working in the rarefied atmosphere of a teaching hospital had given him an appetite for polysyllables, so the notes were liberally scattered with such gems as 'maieusoiphobia' and 'corticopeduncular'. Only when I'd retrieved my medical dictionary, which had been serving as a doorstop in the sitting-room, did I discover that the former meant a fear of childbirth and the latter anything relating to the brain. As the day wore on I discovered, for example, that 'virgynatism' means sexual desire between a husband and wife and 'prosopagnosia' means the inability to recognise familiar faces. 'Thelarche' refers to premature breast development, 'battarism' is a synonym for stuttering and a 'cephalalgia' is a headache.

The second problem I'd been left by my locum did not appear until the very end of the evening surgery. During the day I had examined several patients, asking all of them to undress behind a large old-fashioned screen in a corner of the surgery and then recline upon the couch. As each patient emerged he or she gave me a strange look. The first, Mrs Norton, had come to have her piles examined. She gave me a strange sour look that grew worse when I asked her to lie on her side and pull down her voluminous silken pants. Mr Fraser, who came to have stitches removed from a cut on his leg inflicted by a stone thrown up by his petrol-operated lawn-mower, gave me a conspiratorial wink when he emerged trouserless. And Miss Belcher's eyelids fluttered at twice the usual rate when she came out to have her aching abdomen investigated.

I'd been puzzled by the reactions of all these people but had thought little about them, for the simple but compelling reason that I had other things on my mind. Among the mail on my desk there was a letter from the clerk to the local Family Practitioner Committee, the official body whose job it is to administrate general practice and mediate between doctors, patients and government. Patients pay taxes and national insurance stamps to the Government, which takes a ninety-per-cent service charge and then spends what is left on providing services such as medical care for the people. Although not directly employed by the Government, general practitioners receive their fees from it on behalf of the patients they look after.

The clerk to the Family Practitioner Committee has many functions, but one of his jobs is to deal with complaints made by patients about doctors. In our case he was a pleasant enough fellow, serious, law-abiding and rather cautious. He was the sort of man who, during an electricity shortage, would drive around with dipped headlights in an attempt to be public-spirited. He had, he told me, received a complaint from a Mr Neville which it was his duty to investigate. The complaint was simply that I had failed to take seriously the swallowing of a marble by Mr Neville's son and that the aforesaid marble had, upon passing through the child's gastrointestinal tract, broken the porcelain lavatory pan in the bathroom of the Nevilles' home, causing great distress to all members of the household and damaging their bathroom carpet.

I had never before found myself on the wrong end of an official complaint, but I knew that it had to be taken seriously, bizarre though it might be. The greatest threat to the security of a medical man is the vindictive patient or relative who can cause professional ruin on the slimmest pretext with the aid of the complex machinery provided for that purpose by the profession and the Government.

The laws and regulations concerning the practice of medicine are many, and sometimes bizarre. For example, doctors are not liable to have their horses commandeered to pull fire-engines, but on the other hand they are likely to find themselves in court if arrested for speeding to a dying patient who has requested an emergency visit. The only thing I knew or know about the law is that a doctor can put himself permanently out of a job with his own tongue if he does not seek legal advice speedily. When I received the letter, therefore, my first act was to telephone the Doctors' Defence Group in London and arrange to see a lawyer.

Only later that evening did I remember the curious looks I'd got from the patients who'd changed behind the surgery screen.

Pinned to the screen, I then discovered, was a large colour photograph taken from a calendar produced by a major tyre company. The photograph showed neither a Swiss alp nor an English village scene, but instead a reclining young lady modelling invisible clothes.

26

'TELL ME how you doctors stay fit,' an elderly lady patient of mine had demanded, breathing peppermint fumes into my face one dismal morning when the waiting-room was crammed from skirting-board to picture-rail with coughing, heaving, breathless, germ-sodden citizens.

I had insisted that doctors don't always stay fit and that they, like everyone else, suffer from minor and major ailments. I had discovered that young G.P.s are permanently snuffling. The old lady, however, was not so easily convinced.

'There's some special injection, isn't there?' she had demanded. 'You doctors have a special injection to ward off germs.'

To please her I had finally confessed that all doctors have an injection of secretly made vaccine every year and that, in order to ensure that business booms from time to time, we refuse to share it with the rest of the world. Only then would she depart happily.

I thought about her as I struggled to drag myself out of bed. My head felt as though it had been used as a punchball by the world heavyweight champion, my legs as though they had been replaced by papier mâché replicas. As I sneezed my way into the bathroom I knew that I had the beginnings of a cold.

'Why on earth don't you stay in bed?' asked Margaret, hands on hips, guarding the stairs like a soldier on duty.

'I've got to go to London today,' I reminded her. 'I've got to see this fellow at the Doctors' Defence Group.'

'Damn,' said Margaret with a rare expletive. 'Why can't you just ignore that silly man Neville? He can't be serious. Or, if he is, surely no one *else* will take him seriously.'

'I've got to,' I explained for the tenth time in two days. 'He's charging me with dereliction of duty. I could be struck off the medical register if he proved his case.'

Coughing like a professional I struggled down the stairs, using Margaret as a crutch, and staggered into the kitchen. For a week I'd had a notice hanging up on the front door saying that there would be no surgery that day and that in case of emergency they should telephone Dr Edwards. Despite that I could still hear Miss Williams arguing with a patient who was insisting that he wanted his life insurance examination done immediately.

'Fine example you look,' said Margaret, following me into the kitchen. 'I wouldn't go to a dentist who had toothache.'

I sat down at the kitchen table and put my head in my hands, not in depression but simply because I didn't think I could hold it up without support.

'Can I have a coffee?' I asked.

She busied herself with the stove, making coffee and an omelette.

'I couldn't eat,' I told her.

'You must eat something,' she insisted, 'or else I shan't let you out of this house.'

I muttered something rude about nagging women which Margaret ignored and searched through my pockets looking for the train timetable Miss Williams had collected from the station for me.

'Your timetable is in your inside pocket,' said Margaret, without even looking round. 'And you're catching the 8.45. You've got forty minutes,' she added, examining her watch as she expertly broke another egg.

I replaced my hands underneath my head and waited for breakfast to appear on the table.

There had been a number of advances in the last century. We can fly around the world in hours and send messages in seconds from one hemisphere to the other, we have computers which can do sums in microseconds that men would formerly have puzzled over for years, we can blow each other up simply by pressing buttons and we can put men from this overcrowded planet on to the moon (although, having once done that, we stupidly bring them all the way back again). There have been developments in medicine, too: some diseases have been eradicated altogether, and smallpox for example, is no longer the scourge that it once was.

But many other things have remained the same. The common cold and other simple virus infections are just as annoying now as they have ever been. The first efforts to find a cold cure began in New York in 1926 with Dr Alphonse Dochez and his colleagues. In 1946 the Common Cold Research Unit was set up in Salisbury, England, and since then over 11,000 volunteers have been there to help scientists. Yet we know little more about it now than Dr Dochez did when he started. I suppose our failure is hardly surprising when you realise that even on human skin regularly washed with soapy water and sprayed with deodorants there are probably something like 100,000 microbes on every square centimetre – each a living thing.

'Did you realise,' I asked Margaret, 'that a city of microbes the size of New York lives on the palm of your hand?'

'I really mean it,' said Margaret. 'If you don't eat it, you're not going to London. You need something inside you.'

I'd been married long enough to know better than to stand between a woman and her man's stomach and, besides, the omelette looked appetising. I abandoned a reverie about the number of microbes in all the people in a city the size of Tokyo and ate it.

Two hours later, courtesy of British Rail on one of its better days, I was standing in the middle of New Square in Lincoln's Inn, where many of London's brightest and most expensive legal brains hang their wigs. The Doctors' Defence Group has its offices in one of the largest buildings in the area, a just and reasonable testament to the importance of litigation in medical practice. Research has shown that each doctor is sued every twenty-two months – or that, if most doctors are unsullied by the law, then one is sued much more frequently.

I stood for a moment on the lowest step of the D.D.G. building and stared up at the impressive brass plate above the doorway. Resisting the temptation to pull my collar up lest anyone see me enter the building and assume that I was guilty of some awful crime, I climbed up to the front door. At the top of the steps I paused to sneeze twice, and then approached the smart receptionist who sat at her desk busily filing her nails. I coughed.

She changed hands. She was studying a page of horoscopes with a great deal of interest.

'Excuse me,' I whispered, diffidently taking my letter of appointment from my inside jacket pocket. 'I have an appointment with. . . .'

I looked down at the paper I had in my hand, saw that it was my train timetable and reached in again.

The receptionist abandoned her fingernails, now apparently filed to her satisfaction, and took out a compact which had a mirror in the lid. She began to attend to her face, which seemed to me to need no more repairs than a Rolls-Royce still in the showroom.

'Vernon,' I murmured nervously when I'd found the correct piece of paper. 'Edward Vernon for Mr Lloyd Lloyd-Lloyd.'

'Eleven-thirty,' said the girl absentmindedly. 'I'll show you to the waiting-room.'

Faithfully and sneezing from time to time I followed her along a corridor with a thick and expensive carpet. The walls were decorated with modern prints by the sort of painters who get cross with themselves before they've even started and end up slashing the empty canvas with a sharp knife.

At last we arrived at what was apparently the waiting-room. It was also an office, for a blonde lady in her early twenties sat there at another desk.

I was invited to sit down on a black leather and chromium-plated chair in a corner. A low-slung coffee-table was covered with a thin layer of journals, largely things like the *Solicitors' Journal* and the *Law Gazette*. The Doctors' Defence Group clearly had little idea of the light-reading habits of the rest of the world.

I picked up a two-year-old copy of the *Solicitors' Journal* and began to study the classified advertisements which bore a remarkable resemblance in form and content to those in the *British Medical Journal*. Unable to maintain my interest, I allowed my eyes to wander. The whole room was lined with wooden shelves upon which were stacked rows upon rows of leather-bound law-books and dozens of pieces of folded paper tied up with scarlet ribbon. I assumed that these must be the briefs so beloved of all barristers.

I'd been sitting there for twenty minutes when the telephone rang. The young blonde answered it, spoke briefly to the caller and then came across to me.

'Mr Lloyd-Lloyd has been detained in court. A case from yesterday evening,' she explained. 'He'll be about three-quarters of an hour. Why don't you go out for a walk or a coffee?'

I made my way back down the long corridors and passed the receptionist. She was attending to her eyebrows and studying a crossword without much evidence of interest.

Outside I sneezed again and felt a cough building up inside me. I wandered out of the building and strolled aimlessly among the tourists and lawyers. I kept looking behind me to make sure I didn't get lost when making my way back. I was tempted to carve notches in the more elderly lawyers as they stood around talking. They would, I felt sure, still be in position when I made my way back.

I couldn't find a coffee-shop, but I did find a chemist's. I went in and bought a bottle of linctus to help keep my cough under control. Then I slowly made my way back to the D.D.G. offices. When I walked in through the entrance doors the receptionist was repainting her lips. I walked past her without a word and made my way back to the waiting-room.

Sitting down, I decided to take a dose from my bottle of cough medicine. Having no spoon or glass, I pulled the bottle half-out of its paper bag, so I could swig from it direct. It felt sticky, and I kept the bag around it as I drank.

Just as I had it tilted up to my lips for my second draught the door opened and a tall figure in a black gown flowed into the room. He wore a grey wig, slightly bald at the top, from which a mop of unruly red hair escaped.

'Ll-Lloyd Ll-Lloyd-Ll-Lloyd,' he stuttered.

I stood up quickly, tipping cough linctus down the front of my jacket. I held out my hand to him but apparently that was not the correct form, for he ignored it. It might, I thought, have been the bottle that had put him off. 'Cough medicine,' I said, in explanation, holding it aloft.

Mr Lloyd Lloyd-Lloyd nodded, clearly unconvinced. I half-lifted it from its wrapper, getting my fingers extremely sticky as I did so. Unfortunately my legal adviser had already turned to lead the way to his room. I followed in his wake, having to hurry to keep up with him. My head still felt as if it had been hammered out of shape, and I could feel a whole army of sneezes queueing to get out of my body. I didn't blame them at all.

Mr Lloyd-Lloyd, despite his stern appearance and his stutter, was kind and courteous, though hardly comforting. 'Very serious, very nasty problem,' he said, studying the thick file of papers tied neatly in scarlet ribbon that had been waiting for him on his desk. 'These cases are always nasty.'

'I didn't think it was *that* bad,' I said hesitantly.

'You'll have to plead guilty, of course,' he went on. 'There isn't much point in trying to defend the case.'

'Oh,' was all I could manage.

'I appreciate the fact that it's a worry,' he said, bending forward. 'V-v-very worrying indeed.'

'It is.' I nodded.

'We had a client once who practised in Islington,' he remembered. 'A-a-about your age, if I remember correctly. He was called to see a body in a flat above a fish and chip shop. He certified that the man had died of natural causes, but the undertaker noticed a bullet-hole in the back of the man's head. The insurance company had p-p-paid out by then and they weren't very pleased at all. The policy didn't cover suicide or any sort of violent death. H-h-had a devil of a job getting the poor fellow out of that one.'

'But you did?'

'Well, the Group had to pay damages, but the doctor stayed on the register. So it wasn't too bad.'

'But this case is just about a marble,' I pointed out. 'It really isn't anything too serious.'

'D-o-doesn't have to be serious to be expensive,' he said with a sad shake of his head. 'When there's damage to personal property to be considered there's a principle at stake.'

'Yes, I suppose so.'

'A c-client of ours from Cardiff ripped a stockbroker's j-j-jacket while giving him c-c-cardiac massage,' he went on. 'The stockbroker survived and sued for the cost of a new j-j-jacket. The court was very hard on the d-d-doctor.'

'So I'll have to plead guilty?'

'Easier by far. If you don't, the paperwork will k-k-kill you. And there'll be more meetings than you can stand. We had a c-c-client in Huddersfield whose case d-d-dragged on for three and a half years because he insisted on p-p-pleading not guilty. He'd parked his car in a no-waiting zone and the p-p-police had towed it away. Then he s-s-spent the rest of the morning getting the d-d-damned thing back. It was late afternoon by the time he finished his visits, and one of the patients had d-d-died. He was sued for negligence.'

'What happened?' I asked.

'The case was abandoned after the d-d-doctor got so fed up with it all that he k-k-killed himself.'

'I'd rather it was cleared up quickly.'

'Of course you would,' he said. 'Plead guilty and ask for clemency. We'll look after you. There'll be a disciplinary hearing first and I'll see you at that.' We talked a little more about the size of the marble, the nature of my relationship with Mr Neville, the general health of Mr Neville's son, and my career. Most of the questions I answered, like the cases Mr Lloyd-Lloyd had quoted, seemed to have little bearing on my case. Suddenly it was over. With my mind in a whirl I found myself outside in the corridor. I passed the receptionist, who was filing her nails again, and made my way back to the station. I'd drunk far too much cough linctus and I slept all the way back on the train.

When I got home Margaret told me that there had been a telephone call from the Family Practitioner Committee. Mr Neville had decided to withdraw his complaint.

27

MR BRAND had been getting weaker and weaker for several days. He had insisted from the beginning that I should be truthful about his prognosis and I had therefore had to tell him that I thought his end was very nigh.

'I must know,' he'd insisted earlier on, 'not because my business affairs need putting in order but simply because I want to know where I stand.'

'The truth isn't always as simple as we'd like it to be,' I'd explained. 'It isn't usually possible to say that a patient will last so long with such and such an illness and this long with that disorder. People are all different, and so are prognoses.'

'But you have an idea,' he argued. 'You have a pretty good idea of whether or not I'm going to get any stronger.'

I admitted that I did.

'Then I, too, have a right to know.'

'If you were run over by a bus, or on an aeroplane that crashed, you'd not know,' I pointed out. 'You'd have no chance to prepare yourself.'

'I don't want to know because I think I can solve the problems which my death might bring,' he said. 'I want to know for more selfish reasons.'

I looked at him, hardly understanding.

'I'm a very practical man,' he explained. 'If I'm going to live six months, I shall live differently from the way I'll live if I have a week or six years. If I'm going to get stronger, then I'll go to Athens. I've always wanted to see the Acropolis. If I'm not going to get stronger, then I'll not be able to make it and I'll not bother making plans.'

'You're very calm,' I said. 'People can't always take their impending death so coolly.' I blushed at the word 'death' and cursed myself for using it.

'I've had a good life,' he said. 'I've enjoyed it. I was upset at first when I thought I might be dying, but I've got over that now.'

'How can you get over something so important?' I asked him.

'In time everything becomes bearable as long as you know what's happening. When I was at university I could stand it far better if I'd failed an examination and knew than if I didn't. Knowing made the problem disappear. Instead of being abstract it became a practical problem which could be dealt with.'

And so I'd agreed that he would be told everything of importance. I arranged for Miss Watson the district nurse to call in and help bathe and dress him for as long as he was able to get out of bed. For some time she helped him get ready for work and he'd limp painfully and breathlessly out to the car where the chauffeur would take him into the factory.

'The factory is my life,' he explained. 'If I stay at home all day, what will I do? An early retirement killed my father, and I see men who retire from here dying because they have nothing to live for.'

Hardly anyone at the factory knew that the boss was dying. They knew that he was getting weaker, of course, and that he would sometimes leave early in the afternoon, but most of them merely took that as an example of the rights of the boss to do pretty much as he likes – a right which Mr Brand was probably never aware existed.

'Look after my kidneys well,' he said. 'I've left them and my eyes to your vulture colleagues, and I don't want them to spoil.' I promised him I'd see that his body was taken with all decent haste to the local hospital where it could be frozen preparatory to the arrival of the spare-part surgeons.

He and Miss Watson developed a strong bond. She had something of a reputation for being outspoken and even slightly cruel occasionally. She had what is sometimes known as foot-in-mouth disease. And yet they respected each other. Each had an innate honesty which the other found attractive. Mr Brand, too, had always been blunt and straightforward. Usually he had found himself face to face with the sycophantic dishonesty of fawning subordinates or the critical dishonesty of competitors. Miss Watson, so used to death and dying, had never found the need to develop any sense of what is right and proper. Her boundaries were much more simple ones. She respected the sanctity of death, and of life. In between, she simply said what she thought and expected others to do the same.

As he grew weaker and weaker Mr Brand asked me to stay with him for longer and longer.

'I thought I'd be able to face it without a murmur,' he said, 'but it isn't so easy.'

'You'll not have any pain,' I promised.

'I'll not have you giving me pills and potions to keep me alive,' he insisted. He agreed, however, to let me arrange for Miss Watson or myself to give a regular evening injection of Valium to help him sleep.

'At least it'll give you people a good night's sleep,' he said with a slight smile. 'If I'm asleep, I can't be ringing you up or making a damned nuisance of myself.'

Within a few days, however, it became clear that the Valium was not strong enough to counteract the pain.

'Let me give you something stronger,' I begged him.

'No,' he insisted. 'I'm not dying a damned drug addict.'

I pointed out that I wouldn't let him become an addict and tactfully avoided saying that he wouldn't live long enough for that. He was weaker in spirit as well as in body. Eventually I decided that he must have morphine. Since this is such a dangerous drug I wrote the prescription out deliberately and neatly. I planned to give him one injection a night and others in the day-time as he needed them.

'You're not giving me morphine,' he insisted as I prepared the first.

I started to lie, but couldn't convince him.

'Show me the ampoule,' he insisted. I showed him and ended up giving him another injection of Valium. He slept badly and was clearly in pain. The next night I emptied out a Valium vial before I went into his room, broke open a morphine ampoule and sucked the morphine up into a syringe. I then squirted the morphine into the Valium ampoule.

When I got into his bedroom he checked the ampoule and nodded his satisfaction before I gave him his injection. The next morning he caught my sleeve. 'I slept well last night,' he said proudly. 'You see, I don't need that wretched morphine of yours.'

180

Three days and three injections later he went to sleep one night and never woke. He reminded me a great deal of Mr Campion; one a simple working man with few material possessions, the other a rich factory-owner, but with something of importance in common.

28

THE PRESCRIPTION FOR MORPHINE that I'd written out for Mr Brand had been taken to the chemist's by his mother but not made up without some difficulty. Mr Spencer, the chemist, had telephoned the surgery before handing the ampoules over to Lady Brand.

'Sorry about this, Doctor,' he said. 'Just thought I'd check that you wanted morphine for a Mr Brand.'

'That's right,' I confirmed. 'Couldn't you read my writing?'

'Oh yes,' he said. 'That's just it. It was too legible.' He laughed merrily. 'Your handwriting is nearly as bad as Dr Oaks'.'

'While you're on the phone,' I said, remembering a mental note I'd made. 'Do you have any aminophylline ampoules? I need some for my night bag.'

'Call round any time,' he suggested. 'I'll let you have what you need.'

Evening surgery went fairly well that day, and I'd finished by twenty past six. I went straight round to the chemist's shop and rang the bell.

'I thought I'd just do a little tidying up,' he told me as he unbolted the door. We introduced ourselves to one another and he put a box full of camera films down on the counter.

'Do finish what you're doing,' I told him.

'Well, if you don't mind,' he said, 'I will just finish this window display.' He picked the box up again and carried it over to the window.

'With winter coming on soon,' he said, 'we've got to get the right goods on display. It'll soon be the hot-water-bottle season.'

'I'd never thought of chemists' shops selling seasonal items,' I confessed.

'Oh dear me, yes. Electric blankets in the winter, and sun-glasses and bathing-hats in the summer.'

'I must buy some film,' I remembered aloud.

'I'll let you have some,' he promised. 'I've got some out-of-date stock you can have quite cheap.'

'Well, I don't know . . . ,' I said.

'Oh, it's perfectly all right,' he assured me. 'But it's a few months out of date according to the maker's expiry stamp.'

'Oh,' I said non-committally.

'I tell you what,' he went on, 'you must have lots of drug samples you never use.'

'Well, I suppose I do,' I admitted. 'There are cupboards full of pills I don't ever prescribe and couldn't imagine myself giving away.'

'Well, you bring along your pills,' he suggested, 'and I'll give you a couple of rolls of old film to try.'

'That sounds fair enough,' I agreed.

'Now, you wanted some aminophylline, did you say?' While we'd been talking he'd piled several dozen cartons of film into an expertly designed pyramid which looked as though it would collapse if anyone breathed on it.

'That's right,' I said, 'and a few penicillin injections, too, please.'

'Certainly,' he said. He bustled around behind the counter and put half a dozen ampoules of each into a paper bag.

'How much is that?' I asked him, accepting it.

'Oh, don't let's bother about that. We don't want to bring the tawdry subject of money into the conversation.' He smiled. 'I'll send you a bill.'

'Thank you.' I nodded, not certain that I wouldn't rather pay before I forgot what I'd bought.

'Will you have a drink with us?' he asked suddenly, coming round from behind his counter and scurrying across the shop to a doorway behind the cosmetics counter. 'You must meet my flat-mate,' he said. 'You'll be bound to come across him sooner or later.'

He opened the door as he spoke and disappeared through it. I followed him and found myself in a small courtyard which was full of dozens of pieces of rusting machinery.

'Hobby of ours,' he explained. 'We love old engines.'

I threaded my way behind him through the garden of iron-mongery and eventually found myself clambering up a wooden staircase which led to a door painted black and mounted with a most unusual type of knocker. I couldn't work out what it reminded me of but it wasn't a knocker.

He opened the door and walked into the hall. I followed him.

'Wilfred!' he called. 'Wilfred, I've brought Edward along to meet you.'

I followed him into a large room. The amazing thing about it was that everything in it was white. The walls were covered in the same white fur as the floor and the ceiling, and the furniture was all white-painted wood. Wilfred was not white. He was well tanned and probably in his late forties.

'I'm delighted to meet you,' he said, jumping up and shaking my hand.

'Me too,' I agreed, a trifle uncertainly.

'Wilfred,' said the chemist, 'this is Edward.' He looked at me and smiled affectionately. 'We must be on Christian names, mustn't we?'

'Oh yes,' I agreed. I felt inexplicably uncomfortable.

'Wilfred is an undertaker,' said the chemist. 'And you must call me David.'

'Edward Vernon,' I said, introducing myself.

'Wilfred Davis,' said the undertaker. The introductions promised to continue indefinitely as the chemist shook my hand again.

'A drink?' asked the undertaker eventually.

'Very kind of you,' I said. 'A dry martini perhaps.'

'Oh dear me, no,' said David Spencer. 'We thought perhaps a coffee or cocoa. We don't have alcohol in the flat. Wilfred had hepatitis a year or two ago and we neither of us drink.'

'Not a vice between us,' boasted the undertaker with apparent callous disregard for the truth. He winked at me.

'Do you know a fellow called Pirelli?' I asked. 'He's in the undertaking business, I believe.'

'Do I know him!' cried Wilfred, clapping his hands together in a gesture of dismay. 'Do I know him?' He shook his head rapidly from side to side. 'He's supposed to be one of our drivers,' he said. 'But he's been off work for positively ages. Can't think why. He's as strong as an ox.'

'Well, a coffee would be very nice,' I said.

'Black or white?' asked David.

184

'Black, please.'

'Oh, I can't drink black coffee,' sighed the undertaker. 'I can slip a sherry past my liver at Christmas but I can't get anything past my ulcer.'

'You've got an ulcer?' I enquired.

'Have I got an ulcer?' repeated Wilfred to the world in general.

'He drinks a pint of antacid a day just to keep it satisfied,' said David.

'Still,' said Wilfred, 'there's no future in being a defeatist. The pain gives me the strength for my poetry.'

'He writes a lot of poetry,' said David. 'He had a book of poems out once.'

'Really,' I said, genuinely impressed.

'Didn't sell well,' said Wilfred with a sad shake of the head. 'But it gave away very nicely,' he added with a more cheerful nod.

'What sort of poetry do you write?'

'Modern stuff,' he said. 'Doesn't rhyme, scan or make sense. You know?'

'I know.' I nodded. 'Very good.'

'I don't know if it's very good or not,' he said, taking my comment as a compliment, 'but it does make me feel better. There's no real poetry in dying anymore.'

'Your coffee,' said David, handing me a bone-china cup full to the brim with black coffee. I looked at it and then at the rich white carpet. I took it from him very gently.

'Nearly all go to the crematorium now,' complained the undertaker. 'Just a few bars of a tuneless hymn played on a tape-recorder by an old woman who brings her knitting and presses the button when a red light goes on, and that's it.'

'Bit mechanical,' I agreed. 'Conveyor belt and all that.'

'No worse than pharmacy,' complained David. 'As long as he's tall enough to reach the top shelf and able to count out pills, anyone could be a chemist today.'

'You've just been morbid since you had that operation,' moaned the undertaker. 'Had his piles done last year,' he explained. I sipped at my coffee, holding cup and saucer in both hands.

'Still, we must look on the bright side,' said Wilfred.

'Oh yes,' said David, 'we make a living.'

'Is that what you call it?' asked Wilfred with a wicked smile.

'I really must be going,' I said, looking at my watch and finishing my coffee. I placed the cup down very carefully on a glass-topped coffee-table. It seemed to be suspended in mid-air.

As I left I looked back at the front door. I couldn't see why I hadn't realised it before. The knocker had been made out of a coffin handle.

29

LIKE ALL DOCTORS in general practice I occasionally find myself dealing with patients from other parts of the world. At holiday-time there are calls to see elderly relatives staying for a few days with sons and daughters unaccustomed to the sometimes eccentric demands of the older generation. As we grow old we all grow a little more like ourselves, and often the introduction of an unusually honest member of the family into an already tense situation can produce a minor social explosion with sons, daughters and grandchildren all coming for help.

Sometimes patients from farther afield have appeared in the surgery. Tourists wandering around the country studying old churches and other buildings of note would from time to time pop in to arrange for treatment of minor ailments and illnesses acquired *en route*.

At the beginning of the hay-fever season – earlier that summer – I found the waiting-room almost filled one morning with a group of young Swedish tourists complete with knapsacks and hiking-boots. One after the other they marched into the surgery to ask for pills and sprays with which to control their sneezing and their itching eyes. They told me they'd come to the area to take rubbings from the well-known brasses in a local church.

A German tourist, wearing to my astonishment a pair of leather shorts embroidered with flowers, came into the surgery one day later on, and asked for an appointment to see a plastic surgeon.

'What's up?' I asked him, peering across the desk.

'Cosmetics,' he explained. He leant forward confidentially and nodded very seriously. 'I have wish of becoming more handsome.' He pushed back his hair and revealed, as if by accident, a pair of large pink ear-lobes which stood out at right angles to his head.

'Snip!' he suggested with a snipping motion of his fingers. 'For the girls,' he explained.

'Well, you see,' I tried to tell him, 'this sort of operation cannot always be done under the National Health Service.'

'Cost a great deal of money,' he said with a grim look. 'I cannot afford this at home.'

I began to explain again that such operations were not usually made available to foreigners. He didn't seem to understand. He shook his head vigorously and his ears flapped like sails.

'Let me have a closer look at them,' I sighed.

He grinned contentedly and jumped up. I stood up and began to walk round the desk. To my surprise he unfastened his trousers and let them fall around his ankles. He then slid down his underpants and pulled up his shirt.

'There!' he said triumphantly. He held up his shirt and pointed to his penis.

I scratched my head and stepped back a couple of feet. I idly wondered whether or not the bat-eared German was just a flasher who specialised in doctors' surgeries.

'Snip,' he said. His right hand swooped and picked up his foreskin. 'Snip,' he said again.

'You want circumcising?' I asked him.

'For the girls,' he said again, nodding enthusiastically.

I walked back round the desk and sat down again. The German stood there waving his member at me lest I forget his request.

'You can put it away,' I told him I stood up and pulled up a pair of imaginary trousers. He caught on.

'I'll see what I can do,' I promised.

'Thank you,' he smiled. He wrote down the address of his hotel and handed it to me. 'I'll be there for a week,' he said. He insisted on shaking my hand before leaving. As he did so his enormous ears waved to and fro in time with each other.

Dr Oaks rang that same evening to invite me to a cricket match on my half-day the following week, and I told him about the German.

'Refer him,' said Dr Oaks firmly.

'Refer him?' I repeated. 'But surely it isn't fair to take up

Health Service facilities in providing cosmetic surgery for foreign patients.'

'Of course it isn't,' he agreed. 'But by the time he gets an appointment he'll be back in Germany. You'll have done what you can, but the National Health Service won't have to circumcise him.'

It seemed very obvious when he explained it.

Problems didn't only arise when patients from abroad arrived wanting treatment. Occasionally patients from my practice would receive treatment abroad which would create problems of a different kind. Of course, those falling ill in Majorca or Nice and being treated by the local physician presented little in the way of difficulty apart from translating the explanatory letters accompanying them on return, but there were problems with those who travelled abroad in deliberate search of a cure for a long-lasting ailment. The medical grass always seems greener on the other side of the hill and a few patients, after reading extravagantly worded praise of doctors in clinics abroad, would insist on travelling for treatment, seeking 'magical' cures in Moscow, Switzerland or South Africa.

Mrs Caversham was one such. She read in a women's magazine of a surgeon in Chicago who was said to have developed a wonderful surgical cure for bunions.

'He's tremendous,' she insisted, clutching the article to her bosom. 'He starts at seven and does ten operations every single day of the week.'

I listened with diminishing patience as she explained to me how her hero had banished bunions from the feet of film stars, senators, sportsmen and industrial magnates. My eyelids drooped as she told me how he'd invented a whole range of new instruments made out of platinum with which to perform his operations. Eventually, hypnotised by her dreary voice, I wrote out a short letter of introduction and gave it to her to post to Chicago.

I forgot all about it after that, but a month later she was back. This time she clutched a letter from the great surgeon himself. Well, to be more accurate, it was from the secretary to the assistant to the surgeon himself.

'He's going to do my bunion,' she said in a whisper full of awe. 'He's going to operate on my bunion.' She looked down at her foot and stared at it as if it had suddenly become a holy relic.

The great day was set, and it came too slowly for Mrs Caversham, who appeared in surgery almost daily, desperate to remain healthy enough to travel.

'His operating-theatre is air-conditioned,' she said, 'and I'm sure they'd never let me in with a cold.'

I managed to keep her fit, and eventually the day came for her to leave. She came into the surgery that morning, and I shook her hand and took a long last look at the famous bunion.

I didn't see her again for a month. Then I met her in the local newsagent's when I popped in to buy a new bottle of ink. Like Dr Oaks I used a fountain pen to give my prescriptions a touch of old-fashioned class.

'Good to see you, Mrs Caversham,' I said cheerily.

She seemed not to have heard me.

'Good to see you,' I repeated.

'Oh, hullo, Doctor,' she said without much enthusiasm.

'Back from Chicago?'

'Yes, thank you,' she replied coldly.

'Everything well?'

'Yes, thank you.' She then turned and left without another word.

I discovered later from the district nurse what had happened. Mrs Caversham had slipped while boarding the liner at Southampton and broken her foot in two places. When she'd woken up after the operation the registrar at the local hospital had not only repaired the damage but had also removed the bunion.

30

I COULDN'T SEE MY FEET but I could hear them squelching along in the mud and it wasn't difficult to imagine the damage being done to my brand-new pair of suède shoes. I'd left the car at the entrance to the field partly because I didn't fancy the idea of pushing it out of a pool of mud and partly because the gate was well and truly closed. A huge padlock and a heavy metal chain made it clear that motorised intruders were not welcomed.

'It's a caravan in Sandy Lane,' the woman had said, just before the pips had rudely interrupted our conversation. Before that she'd had time to tell me that she wanted me to visit a friend who had pains in her abdomen and the unlikely name of Crump.

It was raining so hard that the moon hadn't bothered to come out at all and the field was as black as an underground cavern. Black shapes all around loomed like giants; these, I quickly discovered, were all caravans.

Timidly I knocked on the nearest door. A man who must have been well over six feet six inches tall and at least sixteen stone in weight opened it. He looked slightly odd in the doorway with head bowed and shoulders crammed into the tiny opening.

'Excuse me,' I began. 'I'm looking for Mrs or Miss Crump.'

The rain was hammering down so violently on the caravan roof that the giant didn't hear me.

'Eh?' he shouted, cupping an enormous hand about one ear and tipping his head even farther forwards.

'Mrs Crump,' I shouted back.

'No,' he said unnecessarily.

'I'm looking for her.'

The giant nodded.

'Can you tell me where to find her?' I yelled. The rain had

begun to seep underneath the collar of my raincoat and trickle down inside.

'Over there,' he said, waving an arm out into the wet night air.

I followed with my eyes the approximate direction his arm had taken.

'There's a light on,' he said, peering into the darkness.

I looked again and, sure enough, could just discern a glimmer in the distance.

'Thank you,' I called.

'Watch out for the dogs,' he yelled after me.

That stopped me dead in my tracks. Dogs, to my mind, are all beasts of prey. The only dogs I'm not frightened of are the hot ones you eat in bread rolls.

The giant must have seen the look on my face. 'They're on leads,' he assured me. 'Keep in between them and you'll be all right.'

I nodded my thanks and turned back into the bleak and uninviting blackness, keeping a firm hold on my bag, which was the only weapon I had. Caravan sites are not the easiest places in the world to traverse in day-time. Caravan-dwellers seem to have a penchant for littering the land outside their homes with a miscellany of plastic and rubber buckets, tubes and hoses. The grassland on the most organised caravan site is a minefield for the innocent traveller. At night caravan sites could hardly be more dangerous if they were guarded with man-traps.

I found the dogs without any difficulty. It would, perhaps, be more accurate to say that they found me. I was, at the time, busy trying to untangle myself from a washing-line into which I had blundered after treading on a deformed bicycle-wheel that some thoughtless caravandal had abandoned without warning-lights.

Encouraged by two large black dogs of indeterminate breed I managed to extricate myself from the washing-line quite quickly. I then found myself in a predicament. From the left a huge bounding man-eating dog was coming towards me. From the right a second, equally wicked-looking animal was approaching its colleague. There seemed little chance of escape so, like any weak-blooded Englishman, I closed my eyes and began to appeal to the patron saint of dogs to see sense and call off his charges.

People who like dogs offer conflicting advice to those who find them worrying.

'Just keep perfectly still and do nothing at all,' one kind enthusiast will say.

'Bend down and pat them on the head,' says another. 'Any dog will lick your hand if you pat its head kindly.'

'Yell at them with all your might,' say others. 'Scream and shout and make them think you're an even bigger dog. That way you'll frighten all but the most suicidal away.'

Personally I have never found any of this advice the slightest bit useful. When approached by a galloping hound with saliva dripping from its lips and the memory of the taste of human blood still fresh on its palate I instinctively abandon any pretence of reason and prepare to meet St Peter.

This time, after I'd had my eyes closed for what seemed like a decade at the very least, it slowly dawned on me that none of my limbs had been torn from my body. Very slowly and quietly I opened my eyes, wary lest the noise of their opening should attract attention. The two dogs were growling and pawing at the ground no more than a yard away from me. Each had been pulled up by a piece of rope around its neck, and I was just out of reach of both.

I moved forwards slowly, each step taking me farther and farther away from them. A dozen or so steps later I found that they were both well out of biting range. Bravely I smiled at them and even managed to stick my tongue out half an inch.

The caravan with the light on was, naturally enough, on the far side of the field. I reached it some fifteen minutes later soaked to the skin. The door was opened almost as soon as I knocked on it.

'Mrs Crump?' I asked.

'Come inside,' said the woman I'd spoken to on the phone. 'She's on the bed.'

I followed her into the warmth of the caravan.

'Good heavens,' she said. 'What's happened to you?'

I explained that I'd been hiking across the site.

'Oh dear,' she said, genuinely apologetic. 'I should have told you to come along Hornet Lane. There's a gate about twenty yards away that opens on to it.'

I gingerly took off my sopping-wet coat and hung it on the back of the door. Only then did I look around. The inside was extravagantly furnished with miniature reproduction Georgian furniture. A small gas chandelier hung from the ceiling at about chin height. I was clearly in the sitting-room. To my right there was a small kitchen and a shower room. To the left there seemed to be a small bedroom.

'Mrs Crump's in there,' said the woman leading the way. 'I'll stay out here. There isn't room for both of us in the bedroom.'

When I'd squeezed in I could see why. The bed was occupied by the largest woman I'd ever seen, who lay like a stranded whale on top of a pale-blue silk counterpane.

I introduced myself and put my black bag on the floor. Then I sat down on the edge of the bed.

'Where's your pain?' I asked her.

'Here,' groaned Mrs Crump, clapping a hand on her ample abdomen.

I asked her the other usual questions and received no answers worth noting. Asking patients questions about themselves becomes second nature after a while. Only the abnormal answer triggers off any kind of response. Until one is received the doctor continues to fire questions:

'Are your bowels regular?'

'Have you been sick?'

'Have you had this pain before?'

'Are your periods regular?'

'When was your last one?'

'Have you had any trouble with passing water?'

'Have you eaten anything unusual recently?'

'Have you taken any pills in the last day or so?'

And so on.

When I'd exhausted my compendium of suitable questions I began my examination. This promised to be a more than usually arduous task since Mrs Crump's was a larger than usual abdomen. In fact, while sitting on the edge of her bed I could only just reach the far side of it, and when I pressed in deeply to examine the internal organs my hand virtually disappeared, the ocean of fat closing above it like some voracious white sea.

'You're a bit overweight, aren't you?' I asked politely.

'I am,' she said. 'Thirty-five stone eight pound.'

This prompt and unasked-for supplying of information surprised me. Fat patients are usually shy about their precise weight and will generally underestimate by at least ten per cent, just as most patients will underestimate the amount of alcohol they consume and the number of cigarettes they smoke.

My examination of her vast abdomen produced no worthwhile discovery. It was only when I accidentally moved one of her legs that I got a hint as to the actual cause of the problem.

'Do you get pains in your legs?' I asked.

'In my hips and my knees.'

'Is this pain in your abdomen in your back?'

'I suppose it might be.'

From then on it wasn't difficult to discover that what Mrs Crump really had was arthritis. Her unusual size had misled us both. I advised her that she would have to remain in bed and rest a few days.

'You really must try to lose some weight,' I told her. 'You'll get a lot more trouble if you don't.' I explained to her some of the other complaints commonly endured by the overweight, warming to my work as I spoke. Before I left I promised to return later during the day with a diet sheet. Then I got back to the car via Hornet Lane. It was much less of an adventure.

The morning went without incident apart from a visit from Mr Enstone the electrician. Margaret had asked him to fit an extra plug in the kitchen so that we could listen to the radio and make coffee at the same time.

I happened to be in the kitchen with Margaret when he called. We explained what we wanted. To our inexpert eyes, it seemed simple enough. While we sat in silence and watched him he examined the single plug with considerable interest.

'H'm,' he murmured from time to time, for all the world like a doctor examining a particularly unusual bump.

'Is it bad?' we asked him eventually, holding hands under the table for mutual comfort.

'Well,' he said, 'can I look around the house?'

'Yes, of course,' we said at once.

He picked up his bag of tools and walked, shaking his head, from the kitchen into the hall. He examined the sockets in the hall and then moved into the surgery. Having examined the socket and the ceiling fitments there he went into the waiting-room where Miss Williams sniffed loudly when he asked her to switch the fire off for a few moments. All the time, as he worked, he made humming and hawing noises.

'What do you think?' Margaret asked him gingerly, when he'd got back into the kitchen.

'Well, I don't quite know how to put it,' he said, rubbing his chin furiously.

'Tell us the worst,' I begged.

'Well, it's your wiring,' he said, maintaining the suspense with expert ease. 'Did you know about it when you bought the house?' he asked.

'No,' we both shook our heads, almost hysterically.

'It's got no conduit,' he said abruptly.

'No conduit,' said Margaret.

'That's it.'

I didn't know what he was talking about, so I found it difficult to reply.

'And your wiring is all fifteen amps,' he added, clearly feeling that having told us we had a heart condition he might as well add that our blood wasn't in too good a shape, either. It felt strange to be on the receiving end of a gloomy prognosis.

'Is that bad?' asked Margaret.

'Very dangerous,' he said with a shake of his head.

'What should we do about it?' I asked him.

'Rewiring job,' he said. Clearly we were in for major surgery.

'Can you do it?'

'Oh yes,' he said with a firm and comforting nod. 'You're in the best hands.'

'When can you start?' asked Margaret. 'This morning?'

'Oh, good heavens, no, lady.' He laughed. 'Can't do it for ages. Perhaps fit you in in a couple of months if we're lucky.'

'But . . .,' stuttered Margaret. 'If it's dangerous. . . .'

'Oh, it is,' he confirmed, suddenly serious again.

'It's been like this for some time,' I pointed out.

'That's what people always say. You don't know this business like I do. You're lucky to be alive.' He picked up his bag and started for the door. 'Don't suppose you'll be wanting me to put that extra socket in, will you?' he said.

'No,' Margaret said quietly.

When he'd gone I got up and walked across to the kettle.

'Coffee?' I asked. Making coffee is the nearest I get to cooking.

'Yes, please,' said Margaret.

'There's nothing on the radio, anyway,' I pointed out.

My first call after surgery was to the caravan site. I decided to get there early before the rain returned. Even so, I didn't arrive in Hornet Lane till lunchtime, and there seemed to be an extraordinary number of people about. The lane was chock-a-block with people and I could hear the noise of music played at full blast on the other side of the hedge. It was only when I got out of the car that I discovered the caravan site belonged to a travelling fair which was already in full swing for the day.

'I've come to see Mrs Crump,' I announced, after hammering on her caravan door. In my hand I clutched the diet sheet.

'She's at work,' said a small boy with a runny nose and face covered in blood. In his hand he held a hideous thing on a stick.

'What's that?' I asked him, nodding in the direction of the stick.

'Breakfast,' he explained, holding up the wrapper which he had in his other hand and which had clearly covered the lolly a few minutes earlier. 'VEIN ON A CANE,' it screamed. 'FOR VAMPIRES.' 'Want a lick?' he asked.

I rejected his kind offer.

'You're the doctor, aint ya?'

I nodded.

'Mrs Crump asked me to wait here for ya,' he said. He grinned at me. 'You wait till Mr Osborne gets ya.'

I didn't have any idea who Mr Osborne might be, so I walked across to the tent the boy had indicated. As I walked I prepared a suitable admonition for my overweight patient, since when I'd last seen her I'd insisted that she should rest for at least a week.

'You can't come in this way,' said another small boy, guarding the entrance to the tent. 'This is the exit. You go in the front like everyone else. It's 20p.'

197

'I'm Doctor Vernon,' I explained.

He grinned up at me, waved me in with his thumb and whistled shrilly to a colleague fifty or sixty yards away.

Mrs Crump was lying on top of a table draped with bright silk. She wore nothing but a bikini made of identical material. I was struggling through the crowd towards her when I felt a huge hand around my neck. Naturally I stopped.

'You the doc?' asked the owner of the hand.

I would have nodded if I'd been able to.

'What do you mean by trying to put me out of business?'

'Agg Dogg Vugg,' I tried to explain.

'My name's Osborne,' said the man, who was propelling me through the press of people walking past Mrs Crump. 'Wot do ya mean by telling 'er to go on a diet?' We had stopped right beside her and I could now see that the table upon which she lay carried the legend, 'THE FATTEST LADY IN THE WORLD'. I looked around. On the other side of the tent there was a woman with a beard, a dwarf with a head the size of a beach-ball, and the giant I'd spoken to the night before. The giant was busy tearing telephone directories into shreds.

Mr Osborne then propelled me with great vigour back through the crowd and out of the tent.

'Don't come back 'ere,' he called after me.

The small boy who'd announced my arrival winked at me and stepped smartly out of range as I made my way back to Hornet Lane, thoughtfully rubbing my neck. I'd almost reached the exit from the field when the dwarf caught up with me. He carried a goldfish in a bowl and a huge pink teddy bear almost as big as himself.

'Mrs Crump sent you these and says she's sorry for what Mr Osborne did,' he said in an extraordinary high-pitched voice. Then he stood on tiptoe and whispered, 'Have you got that diet sheet?'

I took it out of my jacket pocket and handed it to the dwarf who in turn handed me the goldfish and the teddy bear. Then, carrying these two presents, I made my way back to the car.

31

LIKE EVERY OTHER profession and trade, general practice has been the subject of much close scrutiny from administrators and others dedicated to confusing simple procedures and complicating straightforward tasks. Dr Oaks had apparently found no difficulty in keeping at bay the endless stream of observers and advisers determined to introduce the many varied skills of practice management into his life. As a younger, less well-established and less confident member of the medical profession I found it much more difficult to defend my simple procedures when attacked by the advocates of appointment systems, computerised record-keeping, professional practice management and the medical team.

Innocently, I had in my days as a fledgling doctor imagined that the general practitioner, independent of employer, had responsibilities only to his patients and his conscience. As the first days and weeks of my life in practice went by I discovered that there are many organisations, associations and agencies determined to interfere with the simple and traditional method whereby the patient who feels unwell consults the doctor, who then decides what is wrong and what he or she can do about it. As my career burst into bloom I discovered that there are many people both within and without the medical profession dedicated to destroying such an old-fashioned way of life and adding many complicated and theoretically advantageous clauses to the simple contract which binds doctor and patient together.

Dr Oaks had never in his life seen a patient by appointment. He had held what he referred to as open surgeries. This simply meant that his doors were opened each morning and evening at certain times and closed again an hour or so later. Any patient who was fit enough to leave his home and who wanted advice was expected to present himself at the surgery. Knowing no better, and hoping for nothing more than a life as well organised as that enjoyed by my predecessor, I had followed his example. On some days there were patients queuing up outside, and I would find myself still sorting out their various complaints three hours after I had first put stethoscope to chest. On other days, however – and these were the days which made practice without an appointment system particularly attractive – there would hardly be enough patients to keep me occupied for an hour and a half.

My local colleagues, however, all enjoyed the administrative luxury of properly organised appointment systems. Their days were never unduly busy, but never particularly quiet, either. They had a steady and remorseless stream of patients demanding advice and treatment and, although they never had to endure long and arduous surgeries, they never had the pleasure of light and unexacting ones. When we met occasionally at medical meetings and dinners, the more officious members of the local medical community would all attempt to make me see the error of my ways. Occasionally there would even be protests from patients such as Mr Neville, reared on a diet of socialism and Health Service paternalism and unhappy about waiting for their treatment. When I mentioned these complaints to hardier members of my flock, and suggested that I should perhaps begin an appointment system after all, they would throw up their arms and eyes in horror, mumble about three- or four-day waiting-lists and beg me not to abandon my inefficient antiquated method of practice. I therefore resisted the temptation.

Some suggestions I could not resist, however. One came from the representative of a major drug company who called one day to tell me the good news about his organisation's latest product – a magical preparation designed to diminish the stress of twentieth-century living, prevent heart disease, and cut out strokes, cramp and ulcers of the leg. With some scepticism I listened to his patter, accepted a small library of leaflets, booklets, pamphlets and information-sheets and promised to bear his product in mind should I ever meet a patient whom I felt might benefit from it. This done, the representative produced from his briefcase, with all the flourish of a magician producing a rabbit from his accomplice's coat pocket, a thick pad of sticky labels. Some were red, some were blue and some were green. There were also white ones, pink ones, yellow ones, orange ones, purple ones and violet ones.

'This,' he said, with some pride, 'is our company's contribution to the smoother organisation of your practice.'

I nodded and waited for the explanation which I hoped accompanied the labels.

'Recognising,' he continued in the slightly pompous self-important style of the true company man, 'the importance of an on-going melding of communication skills in the interests of improving the efficiency of the doctor-patient interface, our company has produced these conceptual category guides.'

I looked at him and then at the labels. There seemed to me to be something missing. The representative, apparently noticing my confusion, picked the pad up.

'These category guides,' he went on, holding the pad aloft and peeling a blue label from its backing material, 'are intended to help you distinguish at a glance those patients who need special treatment. These guides will help you create a problem-controlled operation here in your practice.'

I took the pad from him and fondled the half-freed blue label with some care. To me it still bore an uncanny resemblance to an ordinary blue sticky label. I pointed this out.

Shaken, but stirred only to greater oratorial heights, my administrative mentor continued his dissertation.

'We have developed this system,' he told me in a reverential whisper, 'in conjunction with the research department of the British Guild of General Practitioners.'

'Ah,' I said, with an understanding nod.

'As you will know,' he said, 'the B.G.G.P. has — '

'I beg your pardon ?' I asked mischievously.

He looked up suddenly. My interruption was unscheduled.

'The B.G. what ?'

'The B.G.G.P.,' he repeated. 'The British Guild of General Practitioners.'

'Oh yes.'

'We have developed this system in conjunction with the research department of the British Guild of General Practitioners,' he went on. Like all well-rehearsed company men he clearly found that interruptions threw him off his stride and necessitated a fresh start.

'As you will know, the B.G.G.P. has for several years been advocating improvements in the administrative organisation of practice record-keeping,' I was told. 'We have worked with the B.G.G.P. as a service to the profession and jointly prepared these conceptual category guides which we hope you will find a significant service from the B.G.G.P. and Emphatic Laboratories.'

I put the pad of labels down on the desk and stood up. I thought this might suggest to the representative that our meeting had reached its natural conclusion. But he, who had clearly not finished his speech, remained seated and carried on talking.

'The labels are simply attached to the record folders of your patients,' he explained, 'and by their colour they indicate in brief the nature of the patients physical or mental disorder.'

'Some of my patients,' I pointed out, 'have problems that not even a multicoloured rainbow sticker could begin to indicate.'

He was quite undeterred.

'The blue sticker will indicate to you that the patient is a diabetic, the green will suggest that he is left-handed, the violet one will tell you that he is colour blind.'

'So, if a folder has a green sticker, a blue sticker and a violet sticker, it'll tell me that the patient's a colour-blind left-handed diabetic?'

'Exactly!' he cried, thumping the desk so hard that my fountain pen rolled on to the floor. As I was standing up, I failed to catch it.

'The whole chart of colour symptom indices is printed in here,' said the representative, handing me a leather wallet which he produced with his usual flair from his inside jacket pocket. 'You will see,' he said as I opened it, 'that we call this the conceptual category guide key.' He then stood up. He had clearly decided that the interview had finally come to a close. We bade each other brief goodbyes and, realising that the evening surgery was ten minutes late in starting, I pressed my buzzer straight away, diving under the desk as I did so to search for my pen.

From my vantage-point on the carpet I could clearly see the

first patient as he marched into the surgery. He carried a bicycle pump and still wore his bicycle clips.

'Good evening,' I said. 'Please sit down.'

The patient halted two feet inside the room and looked round him in horror.

'Sit down,' I said. Suddenly I spied my fountain pen. I picked it up, backed out from underneath the desk and stood up. The patient's eyes grew larger and seemed about to fall out of his head.

'I didn't see you there,' he drawled in the slow speech of a countryman.

'Lost my pen,' I explained.

The patient said nothing but edged into the room with a little more confidence.

'Do sit down,' I said.

He still looked nervous. He clearly wasn't used to finding his medical adviser hiding underneath the surgery desk. I tried to put him at ease. 'Have you come far?'

'Six miles.'

'That's a fair bicycle ride,' I commented. 'I couldn't ride that far unless it was all downhill.'

'How did you know?' he asked in a terrified whisper.

'How did I know what?'

'How did you know I came on me bicycle?'

'The pump,' I said, pointing. 'And the cycle clips.' I pointed to his trousers, neatly folded inside them.

'You're an observating man,' he said with a grin of appreciation. He shook his head in some disbelief and sat himself down.

'What can I do for you?' I asked.

'I've been low.'

'Low?'

'I don't have an inferior complex, Doctor,' he said earnestly. 'I just am inferior.'

'That's bad.'

'Oh, it's bad.' He nodded. 'It's bad.' He told me he'd been feeling low for several weeks. I asked him why he hadn't been to see me before. He told me he'd felt sure he'd feel better in due course. I asked him how he slept. He told me he didn't sleep well. It didn't take an observating man to see that he was severely depressed.

'What's your job?'

'I'm a woodman. I work in the forest. I like trees,' he said.

'So do I,' I told him.

'We're losing a lot. Chopping,' he explained. 'Elms.'

'They've got Dutch Elm Disease?'

'That's it,' he nodded. 'I hate it. We had a lot of lovely elms. Lost a hundred and fifty this month.'

We talked a little longer and then I prescribed a course of antidepressant pills. I told him I wanted to see him again in two weeks' time and before he went I looked at my conceptual category guide key. I thought it might be a good idea to try it at least. I saw that the white sticker was the one intended for use on the folders of those patients suffering from depression. I therefore peeled one off and applied it to the outside of his notes. He then went, clutching his prescription.

The next patient appeared with his wife.

'Mr Bill Lynn,' said a stern-looking woman in a hat and a flowery print dress which contained all the ingredients for a fruit salad apart from the cream.

'Mr Lynn,' I said, looking at her and then at the rather wizened figure who had accompanied her into the surgery.

'My name is Maude Lynn,' she said, playing with the clasp of her handbag, shaking her head and looking down her nose as if anxious to dislodge some foreign object from its tip. As she shook her head the fruit swung from side to side. 'My Bill's had his operation.'

'Oh,' said I. 'I'm sorry. I don't remember. . . .'

'You were off on your holidays. There was another gentleman here.'

'Oh yes.' I smiled. 'The locum.'

'I thought he was a doctor,' she said with a frown.

'He was.'

'Hmph,' she snorted. 'He said our Bill had a swelling,' she added.

'And he's had it repaired?'

'Hmph,' she snorted again. 'Your Dr Locum said that in two months my Bill would never know he'd had the operation, didn't he, Bill?'

Bill nodded meek agreement.

'When did he have it?' I asked.

'Six weeks ago,' she said.

I nodded and waited for her to continue.

'Never know he'd had the operation,' she repeated.

'That's right.' I smiled professionally.

'Hmph,' she snorted for the third time. The fruit seemed about to abandon hat.

'Isn't it healing?' I asked her. Somehow Bill seemed about as essential to the conversation as his wife's hat. It was not easy to remember that we were talking about him.

'Show him,' said Mrs Lynn. It was an order, not a request.

Mr Lynn duly unfastened his trousers and lowered them, with his underpants to his ankles.

'Look!' said Mrs Lynn, pointing with trembling finger to her husband's groin. The normal landscape was spoilt by a large clearly defined hydrocele – a fluid-filled swelling in the scrotum.

'Said he'd never know he'd had the operation in two months,' she said with another hmph. '*Six weeks* and he doesn't know he's had it!'

'Sometimes . . .,' I began, in an attempt to explain away the disaster.

'Cover it up, Bill,' said Mrs Lynn. She waited, arms crossed, while her husband obeyed.

'Hmph,' she said with a final wave of her cherries. 'Come on, Bill.'

Her husband, who hadn't spoken a word, left in his wife's wake.

I was still pondering the relationship between Mr Lynn, his wife and his hydrocele, which seemed to me to merit the technical term 'ménage à trois', when the next patient appeared in the surgery. I must have pressed the buzzer automatically. I was somewhat surprised to see that it was none other than Mr Neville.

'Good evening, Doctor,' said my audacious persecutor.

I managed a semi-frozen smile.

'No hard feelings, I hope,' he grinned.

I found it difficult to think of anything suitable to say. But Mr Neville didn't want to give me time.

'I've got a list,' he said, pulling out a list as long as a wooden leg. 'A few little problems.'

'I really think,' I began, struggling hard to remain cool and unemotional, 'that it might be better if you found a different doctor.'

'No need for that,' he said with a graceful smile. 'No hard feelings. All forgotten now. We don't bear any grudges.'

I opened my mouth, but the words I'd aimed in its direction failed to appear. I think they probably felt too embarrassed to appear in public.

'I think I've got a varicose vein coming,' he went on, standing and pulling up his left trouser-leg.

'They can kill you,' I told him. 'You'd better see someone else about that.' I scribbled a note.

'Little rash behind my ear,' added my most unwelcome patient.

'Skin specialist,' I murmured, making another note. 'I know a good man in Liverpool.'

'Bit of constipation.'

'Barium enema and gastroenterologist,' I muttered as I scrawled. 'There's a marvellous fellow in Glasgow.'

'You can deal with these little problems,' he said with a smile and a wink.

I shook my head. 'Specialist for you every time,' I said. 'I'll fix up the hospital appointments.'

'I'll be spending all my life at the hospital,' he protested.

I shrugged.

His smile disappeared.

'I'll complain,' he snapped.

'What for?' I asked him. 'You can hardly complain that I'm getting you specialist care for all your problems.'

He said nothing more but to my intense relief walked out of the surgery. I hoped that he would never walk back in.

The telephone rang before I could buzz again. It was the woodman, calling from a telephone box.

'Sorry to bother you,' he apologised. 'How many of these pills do I need to take?'

'Just two at night,' I told him.

'No,' he said, 'to do the job properly.'

'That's all you need.'

'Then why did they give me so many of them?'

'Two at night for two weeks,' I told him. 'They should have given you twenty-eight pills.'

There was silence for a moment. Then he confirmed that the chemist had indeed given him twenty-eight pills. 'I want to get it over with,' he went on.

I felt a chill of horror.

'What do you mean?'

'I saw the white label,' he said.

'White label?'

'I'd rather get it over with,' he repeated.

'Can you come back to the surgery?'

'When?'

'Straight away.'

'I'm only just along the road.'

'I'll be waiting for you,' I promised. I went to the front door as soon as I heard the telephone click and waited for him to appear. Not until I saw his bicycle did I breathe at all easily again. When he'd settled in the surgery I asked him why he'd suddenly become determined to get it over with. 'You didn't feel like that when I spoke to you before, did you?'

He shook his head.

'What happened?'

'The white label,' he said. 'I know what that means.'

He explained that when a tree was too badly diseased to save they put a white mark on it. The white mark meant that the tree was doomed. Seeing me mark his folder, he had been convinced that I had decided that he, too, was doomed. I explained to him what the white mark really meant and then peeled it off his folder and threw it into the waste-paper basket. That seemed to cheer him a little. He promised to return in a fortnight's time.

When he'd gone I gave the sticky labels to Margaret. She said she'd use them to label tins in her storecupboard. I told her she'd be the only housewife in town with a conceptual category-guided larder.

32

ACCORDING to ecologists and conservationists, many of the creatures we love most will soon be extinct unless we do something to help them. The panda, the koala bear, the eagle and many other varieties of fowl and flesh are being herded out of existence by their bipedal cerebrating superior.

Much as I love and enjoy the existence of such rarities, I am more concerned about the likely disappearance of a creature far more essential for a comfortable and contented life. It is the disappearance of the traditional and long suffering 'wife' that future generations may mourn with genuine feeling.

Fortunately Margaret did not seem in the slightest to mind being married to a fine example of the variety of hog so widely and repeatedly disparaged by those feminists who believe that a woman's place is as far away from the home as possible. Bra-burners may find sock-washing, shirt-ironing and stomach-filling tedious, but socks have to be washed, shirts have to be ironed and stomachs, particularly mine, need filling regularly.

As the wife of a general practitioner Margaret had to put up with considerably more than this, however. Not only did my patients regard her as being their property as much as mine, but she was also expected to play a part in local social life. She was invited to become a member of the Women's Institute, the Church Bazaar Committee and the Wives' Discussion Group. Dutifully she joined. It was a request which came in November that year which very nearly frightened her into flight.

The call was from Mrs Bridmarsh, the churchwarden's wife, who was also chairman of the Winter Fayre Committee.

'I'm so sorry to put upon you so suddenly,' said Mrs Bridmarsh, to Margaret, in a tinny screechy voice that very nearly obviated the use of the telephone altogether. I could hear her quite clearly.

'What can I do?' Margaret asked her, probably thinking she

was about to be recruited to bake cakes or produce a donation for the fancy-goods stall.

'Mrs Dewhurst, the vicar's wife, was going to open our Fayre for us,' said Mrs Bridmarsh, 'but unfortunately she's gone down with laryngitis. It's most dispiriting.'

'Oh dear,' said Margaret, 'I am sorry to hear that.'

'The vicar says there isn't a chance of her being well enough to open the Fayre. So my committee and I wondered if you would be kind enough to do us the honour?'

Margaret suddenly paled. I pushed a chair behind her quickly. She sat down.

'Shan't want you to make a long speech or anything, my dear,' said Mrs Bridmarsh. 'Just a few words about how nice it is to be there and how hard everyone has worked. You know the sort of thing. Keep it fairly regal.'

'Oh, I couldn't. I really couldn't.'

'Nonsense,' said Mrs Bridmarsh. 'You were coming, weren't you?'

Margaret admitted that we had both hoped to call in.

'Then there's no earthly reason why you can't,' insisted Mrs Bridmarsh. 'We'll all be most awfully honoured.'

'Oh dear,' was all that Margaret could manage.

'And we'll want you to judge the cakes,' Mrs Bridmarsh added. 'Just pick the winner of the five-pound grocery voucher.'

'Oh no,' cried Margaret. 'How can I do that?'

'Just take a nibble at them all and decide which one you like best,' said Mrs Bridmarsh. 'Mrs Hutton, Mrs Jones or Mrs Tomkins usually wins.'

When Margaret put the telephone down she looked as if she'd just been sentenced to death. 'Can't you say that we've been called away to an important conference in Moscow?' she begged me.

I told her that I was on call that weekend and that everyone would know it.

'Well, can't I have laryngitis or something?' asked Margaret.

I had to point out that it might look suspicious.

Fortunately for both of us the Fayre was due to take place two days later, and the burnt collars and singed bacon which undoubtedly resulted from Margaret's nervous state promised to be over before my wardrobe or stomach could be exhausted.

The Fayre had been organised with little regard for the weather. Hopeful, perhaps, that holding it in the grounds of the church hall would provide immunity from elemental furies the committee had organised a number of outdoor competitions and several dozen outdoor stalls. At ten on Saturday morning, when I took Margaret along for a look at the arrangements, several dozen enthusiastic helpers were busily struggling in what seemed like a force-nine gale to put up canvas-roofed stalls.

As we walked around Margaret rehearsed her speech. At least twenty times I assured her that it was quite perfect, and at least twenty times she told me that she was convinced that she would end up the laughing-stock of the entire town.

'I bet I fall off the dais just as the man from the local paper is taking his wretched photograph,' she insisted.

Her state of mind was not improved by meeting the Rev. Dewhurst and his wife. They, too, were busily involved in helping to put up a stall.

'Good morning, Mrs Vernon,' said the vicar's wife with a distinct croak in her voice.

'Good morning,' said Margaret rather coolly.

'It's so good of you to stand in,' said Mrs Dewhurst, 'I couldn't possibly say a word with this voice of mine. It's almost completely disappeared twice today.'

'Are you really sure you can't manage it?' asked Margaret.

'Absolutely,' said the vicar's wife. She patted Margaret on the hand and leant forward confidentially. 'You mustn't disappoint Mrs Jones,' she said. 'She's really looking forward to winning the cake competition.'

'I hope we have a good turnout,' said the vicar. 'People do tend to stay at home and watch the television a lot these days.'

'Some of them would watch the interference if there were nothing else to watch,' his wife confided to me.

'I'm having a bird's nest guessing competition,' said the vicar. 'You have to guess how many pieces there are in a nest, then afterwards we'll take it apart and find out who is closest.'

'Fascinating,' I agreed.

Mrs Dewhurst caught sight of the choirmaster's wife and excused herself before hurrying off. Margaret was captured by

Mrs Bridmarsh, who began to explain to her just why Mrs Hutton ought to win the cake contest.

'I had that thing removed,' whispered the vicar, leaning close and spluttering in my ear.

'Er . . . good,' I said.

'I can wear short-sleeved shirts now.'

'Splendid,' I said. I still had no idea what he was talking about.

'My tattoo,' said the vicar, realising my confusion.

'Ah,' I said. 'That's marvellous!'

'Sh,' he said. 'Top secret.' He winked.

I winked back, plucked Margaret away from Mrs Bridmarsh and took her home for lunch.

Her speech at the opening was a tremendous success and she faltered neither in speech nor step. A boy who wore shoes like dodgem cars and a plastic mackintosh that reached right down to his ankles presented her with a bouquet of rather bedraggled-looking yellow roses and they both stood together in the light rain for a few frozen moments while the photographer for the local weekly newspaper struggled to take the requisite picture to immortalise the moment.

We were watching a group of fathers manipulating kites in a competition to find the best kite-flier under 12, and waiting for the dreaded moment when Margaret would find her diet abandoned for a hectic half-hour while she was busily tasting cakes when the vicar rushed over to tell me that there had been a call for me to go to an address in the centre of the town.

Giving Margaret a good-luck squeeze I scurried off to do the visit and get back if possible in time to rescue her from any offended bakers. The town centre was very quiet. One could actually park one's car in some of the streets, and I slid gratefully into a space only a few yards from the address I'd been given.

Number 65 Day Street turned out to be a brightly painted green door decorated with a smart, highly polished brass plate upon which were inscribed the words 'Featherweight Slimming Clinic'. I thumbed the white plastic bell below it. A moment later an extremely pretty girl came to the door.

'I'm Doctor Vernon,' I said. 'I hope I haven't come at an inconvenient time. There was a call.'

'Oh, come in, Doctor,' said the girl. 'I'm Jane.'

'Thank you,' I said, following her inside. The front door shut silently behind me. The carpet was soft and clearly expensive, and the corridor itself looked long enough for indoor athletics.

'Here we are,' said Jane finally, coming to a halt outside a bright vermilion door. She knocked a couple of times and then opened it.

'Dr Vernon,' she said, before disappearing back down the corridor. I walked in, not knowing what to expect.

'Hullo!' said a well-preserved woman in her mid-forties. She had an excellent figure which was well exhibited by a smart green jumper and skirt. 'I'm Mrs Crump.'

'Hullo,' I said, shaking her hand. 'You have a problem?'

'That's right,' she said. 'Thank you for coming. One of our customers has fallen and hurt himself. I don't think there's any serious damage, but I'd be very grateful if you would have a look at him.'

'Certainly.'

'You don't recognise me, do you?' said Mrs Crump, standing directly in front of me. She was half-laughing.

'I'm afraid I don't,' I confessed. The name meant nothing to me. 'I've really got a dreadful memory for faces.'

'You must meet an awful lot of people,' she said kindly.

I mumbled something about that not being a proper excuse.

'When we last met I weighed rather more than I do now,' she said with a beaming smile. 'It was at the fair.'

'The Fayre?' I said, confused for the moment with the event I'd just left. Then it came to me. 'You were....'

'The fat lady!' she said. She picked up a folder from the desk and flicked it open. It contained several large colour photos of a very fat woman. It was difficult to believe that this was the same Mrs Crump standing in front of me.

'I left the fair and decided to set up a slimming clinic,' she went on. 'I had some money saved.'

'Fantastic,' I said, meaning it.

'We're only just starting really, but there seems to be a demand.'

'What sort of things do you do?'

'Oh, we have exercise classes and diet discussions, and we sell slimming foods,' she told me. 'I'm having a dieters' restaurant built upstairs.'

'Who's injured, then?' I asked.

'We have a massage parlour,' she explained. 'Some of our customers think they're entitled to rather more than a massage.'

'I'm not altogether surprised,' I said, 'having just seen one of your girls.'

'Well, we don't mind them looking, but our girls are like doctors really. They're encouraged to regard people's naked bodies as simply needing treatment. We don't allow them to become emotionally involved with clients.'

'What happened?'

'One of our slimmers tried to get fresh with Daphne,' said Mrs Crump. 'She put up with a few tweaks. Most of our girls get their bottoms pinched and take it in their stride — '

' — like housemaid's knee or tennis elbow?' I suggested.

'If you like. But after a few tweaks she gave the client a slap. She hit him rather too hard and he fell off the massage table.'

'Is he hurt badly?'

'Mainly his pride, I think. But I'd appreciate your having a look at him.'

I followed her farther along the corridor and into a steamy room where there were half a dozen massage tables, each in a separate cubicle. On one table I saw a face I recognised.

'Hullo,' I said, cheerily. 'It's Councillor — '

'This is the customer who fell off the table,' said Mrs Crump.

I don't know who was more embarrassed, Councillor Wells or I. I examined him, found no signs of damage apart from some slight bruising, and suggested that he get dressed.

'Can I go home?' he asked.

'Yes.'

'I don't have to have any X-rays?'

I shook my head.

'You, er . . . won't, er. . . ?'

'Professional confidence,' I assured him.

'Thursday next?' the Councillor said to Mrs Crump as he pulled his trousers on.

'On condition you remember that the girls are not to be molested,' said Mrs Crump, rather like a schoolmistress.

'I apologise for this afternoon,' he said.

I left them and hurried back to the Fayre.

When I got there Margaret was beaming like a cat who has found a half-full carton of cream.

'All right?' I asked her breathlessly.

'Fine,' she said.

'How did it go?' I hissed.

'Thank you so much, Mrs Vernon,' said a woman in a tweed coat and a feathery hat. She shook Margaret's hand and moved on.

'Who was that?' I asked.

'Mrs Hutton,' answered Margaret, just as a woman in a blue gaberdine mackintosh appeared and said much the same thing.

'Mrs Jones,' said Margaret in reply to my unasked question. Mrs Bridmarsh was next to come and congratulate her. Then came the vicar's wife.

'I think you made a very wise decision,' said Mrs Dewhurst. 'I do hope you can come to our January Festival.'

'I shall be delighted,' said Margaret.

'What have you done?' I muttered, frantic with curiosity.

'I awarded the prize for the best cake,' said Margaret. 'That's all.'

'How did you manage to keep them all happy?' I demanded.

Just then Mrs Young came over towards us, helped by her husband and the district nurse.

'Hullo,' I said, assuming that she'd come to greet me.

'Hullo, Mrs Vernon,' she said, patting Margaret's hand. 'Thank you. You've really made my day.'

I looked at them both.

'Your wife gave me the prize for the best cake,' said Mrs Young proudly. 'It's the best convalescent present I could have.'

'Very canny,' whispered the district nurse. 'Mrs Young is very popular. Everyone knows she's been poorly and just come out of hospital.'

'How did you do it?' I asked Margaret when they'd all gone.

'Do what?' she replied in apparent innocence.

'Decide to give Mrs Young the prize?'

'Her cake was the best,' answered Margaret, quite open-eyed.

214

33

'YOU'RE QUIET this morning,' I said to Margaret as I reached for a third piece of toast and began to smear it with a thick layer of chunky marmalade.

'You've not put butter on that, have you?' she asked, looking up from the magazine she was reading.

I shook my head.

'There's a report here that claims that doctors live to an average age of only sixty-three.'

'That's a cheerful start to the day,' I commented, taking a bite of my toast.

'It says they don't look after themselves as well as they look after their patients,' she continued, 'and according to these figures you'd live longer if you were a clergyman or a school-teacher.'

'But I'm not,' I argued. 'Do you want some more coffee?'

'You're not to have more than one cup,' she said, putting a hand on my arm as I stood up to fetch the percolator.

'Why on earth not?'

'Black coffee is bad for you.'

I laughed. That was a mistake.

'This is very serious,' she said, looking very serious. 'You've got responsibilities now; you're a married man.' She looked at me and brushed a crumb or two of toast from my moustache. 'Besides,' she added, 'I love you.'

'Is that why I can't have butter on my toast?'

'Butter is very bad for you. You should know that.'

'I hope you're not going to start feeding me from that dread-ful health-food shop,' I mumbled, munching the remains of my toast. 'I like salads, nuts and rice, but I like steak and malt whisky as well.'

'And you've got to start taking more exercise,' she said, putting her magazine down firmly. 'You hardly do any physical exercise at all.'

'I'm not running round the park every evening,' I said. 'And I know why long-distance runners are lonely.'

'Why?' she asked, puzzled.

'They smell of sweat and wintergreen.'

'A lack of exercise is one of the factors responsible for heart attacks and high blood-pressure,' said Margaret, who'd picked up her magazine again.

'I *do* exercise,' I protested. 'I walk to the car every time I go out, and hammering people's knees is hard work.'

'That's not the right sort of exercise,' she said, obviously unwilling to give in.

'Well, what do you want me to do?' I sighed.

'I don't know,' she confessed. 'Take up squash, for example.'

'A dangerous activity,' I warned her. 'I heard of a man who dropped dead in the changing-rooms after a game of squash and I can't remember how many people I've seen with damaged eyes and bruised limbs after they've been hit by a squash ball or racket.'

'Well, golf, then.'

'Golf is risky, too,' I argued. 'The exercise is really hardly worth having and there's the very real danger of becoming an alcoholic at the nineteenth hole.'

I dismissed her next idea, table tennis, by recounting the story of a medical student friend of mine who'd broken a leg leaping the net after winning a game.

She then proposed that I take up tennis. I pointed out that tennis balls travel at something over one hundred miles an hour when hit properly. She suggested that I take up sailing or swimming. I pointed out that drowning is an important cause of death in young adults. She said she thought I was just being awkward and obstructive. I suggested that I might take up bridge. She said I was being facetious.

At this stage I looked at my watch and discovered that the morning surgery should have started ten minutes before.

'I shall have to go,' I said, standing up.

'Not until you've promised me that you'll start exercising.'

'Think of something suitable,' I told her, moving away from the table with another piece of toast in my hand.

'You could always take up weight-lifting or buy some equipment for exercising at home,' she said, rescuing the piece of toast.

I licked the crumbs from my moustache.

The argument continued at lunch-time.

'You can't expect your body to remain in good working order unless you look after it,' Margaret began as she poured some asparagus soup.

I pointed out that the human body is by no means incapable of looking after itself and that when buffeted by environmental hazards it has a tendency to rock back into position like one of those dolls with lead-filled bases.

'You can't argue with the statistics,' she said, firmly putting a small piece of cheese and three lettuce leaves in front of me.

'I'll have my soup first,' I said, resisting with some difficulty the temptation to point out the doubtful value of statistics.

'This is all I think you should have,' she said, pointing to the cheese and lettuce. She sat down and began to eat her asparagus soup. I adore asparaus soup.

'Why?' I asked. 'I've been working hard this morning.'

'If you won't take exercise, I shall have to make sure that your body only gets the food it really needs.'

'It needs asparagus soup.'

'You may think it does, but it'll be much happier with something lighter.'

I explained that the human body knows best what food it needs and that my body had decided it wanted something more substantial than a reluctant cheese salad.

'Then will you promise to get some body-building equipment?' she asked. 'And stuff for exercising at home?'

I looked at the asparagus soup and sniffed the steak and kidney pie in the oven. I nodded, and I must say that at the time I thoroughly intended to keep my promise and take up some form of exercise. Although I would never have admitted it to Margaret, I did rather fancy the idea of owning a muscled body suitable for beating off sandcastle bullies. The prospect of building and maintaining a trouble-free frame within which my spirit could roam undisturbed was attractive – particularly since it did seem to me that it would be painless and comfortable to do the necessary exercises in my own home.

What both I and Margaret had overlooked is the fact that the human body is rather like any other piece of complex machinery in that, left alone to its own devices, it may function perfectly happily but that, when subjected to interference from well-meaning mechanics, it will in all probability suddenly develop a hundred and one unexpected faults.

I acquired some equipment from Mr Gladwyn, a patient who had strained his shoulder muscles trying to cram a seven-week body-building course into the three days before his summer holidays. He was happy to sell me his whole collection, including an exercise bicycle which could be pedalled at over forty miles an hour without any need for waterproof cape or lights, at half-price.

'You wait and see,' said Margaret fondly as I dragged the huge box into the house. 'You'll be glad you took my advice.' Stupidly I accepted her forecast and innocently ignored the experience of Mr Gladwyn.

'No dieting?' I asked her as I toyed idly with the chest-expander.

'No dieting,' she promised.

'I can eat what I like?'

'You'll be using up as many calories as you eat. There's no reason at all to restrict your intake.'

That was enough for me. I pulled off my shirt, flexed all the muscles I could find and began to pull at the chest expander.

The accident which followed did not put me off exercising completely, but it did dampen my enthusiasm. I'd extended the heavy steel springs almost to their limit when I suddenly felt myself quite unable to hold them any longer. I let go. Relieved of the pressure from my muscles, the springs shrank back to their original size. The problem was that as they shrank they caught hold of the hairs on my chest.

Margaret said afterwards that she thought I'd exaggerated and that my screams were unnecessary. I still disagree, as I did at the time. I pointed out to her that, had our positions been reversed, she, too, might have felt the need to make some sort of vocal protest.

'Stick to the weights and the bicycle,' she suggested. 'Abandon the chest expander until you're a better match for it.'

This seemed a good idea, so I put the chest expander in a safe place, whence it would be unlikely to escape and damage anyone else, and began to put together the weights. I had no idea just how many weights to fit on to the bar to start with and so I compromised by putting on just the smallest of the seven available metal discs. It seemed unlikely that I would be able to do any damage with such a small weapon.

I was pleasantly surprised to find that I could lift the bar and weights quite easily. I lifted it above my head, lowered it to my waist and began to lift it up again. I'd got it to head height for the second time when the right-hand weight fell off.

The noise didn't sound too bad in the bedroom where I was exercising, but it must have sounded devastating down below, for Margaret came rushing up the stairs at an enormous speed.

'What's happened now?' she demanded breathlessly.

I pointed to the weight on the floor, and slowly put the bar and remaining weight down on the bed.

'One of the chandeliers my mother bought us for our wedding has fallen from the ceiling and smashed.'

'I just picked it up like this,' I said, lifting the bar off the bed, 'and the damned thing fell off.'

At this, the other weight fell off. This time I heard the crash down below.

'That's the other chandelier,' cried Margaret, hurtling out of the bedroom and back down into the living-room.

Slowly I put the empty bar down on the floor and followed her.

'I don't think I'm cut out for exercise,' I said quietly.

'You're supposed to fasten the weights on,' she said, picking up some of the pieces of chandelier which were scattered all over the carpet. 'I give up. You'll just have to stay unfit.' A tear slid down one cheek.

I put my arm around her and kissed it away.

'If I didn't know you better,' she said, wiping her eyes with a handkerchief, 'I'd think you'd done that on purpose.'

I kissed her again. 'There is one type of exercise I like.'

'What's that?' asked Margaret.

I kissed her again. This time on the lips.

Margaret said something, but I didn't quite catch what it was.

34

SUDDENLY it was Christmas. My first year as a fully fledged, if slightly unsteady, general practitioner was nearly over. I found it difficult to believe that it was two years since I'd first met Dr Oaks, Miss Williams and the great variety of patients whose health had become my responsibility. That responsibility seemed an intolerable burden when considered coldly and scientifically; only when accepted on a day-to-day basis was it bearable. Only then did the problems seem simply down-to-earth and practical.

For weeks before the festive day itself the shops had all been busily promoting their seasonal wares. The supermarkets had filled their windows with details of special offers for plum puddings, frozen turkeys and all the delicacies from foreign lands which are for some reason fashionable at Christmas. Nuts, dates and olives crowded the windows alongside oranges and succulent raisins.

Bowled along by the spirit of goodwill and good cheer to all men including shopkeepers, I had stopped at a corner shop near the surgery on the way home from a particularly tedious visiting-list and bought an enormous Christmas tree, so vast that three feet of it had hung out of the back of the car. As a warning to following motorists I had tied my tie (a garish red in colour) to the very tip. Buying it had been a hazard in itself. The shop-owner, a red-faced fellow with a richly veined nose and the smell of good whisky on his breath, swayed precariously as I made my choice from the forest which filled his shop. Eventually I'd thrust the two pounds he'd asked for into his hands and picked up a particularly green and healthy-looking conifer.

When I got back home Margaret was out and Mr Davis the undertaker was sitting in the surgery waiting. He had a cremation certificate ready for me to sign. Mr Hodgson, a ninety-seven-year-old retired milkman who'd been ill for a week with pneumonia, had died the night before, and the undertaker had brought both certificate and fee with him. One of the paradoxes of medical practice is that the fee a doctor gets for signing a cremation certificate when a patient dies is approximately three times as much as he has received for looking after the same patient for a year.

'Like it!' said the undertaker with a wink when I entered. 'Not seen one that big for a long time,' he added. 'It looks strong and firm. It ought to stand up straight.' He walked around the tree and me. 'Good colour too. Look nice with some brightly coloured balls on it and a fairy on the very tip.'

I put the tree down in a corner of the hall and took the form from him.

'Party on Christmas Eve,' he said as I signed my name at the bottom and accepted the small rustling brown envelope with practised reluctance. 'Would you and your good lady like to come?'

'Very kind of you,' I said.

The pre-Christmas surgeries were unusually busy as patients rushed to get their prescriptions signed and dispensed before the holiday. And then two or three days before the day itself things became quieter than I had ever known them.

'It's always quiet just now,' explained Miss Williams. 'They're all too busy doing last-minute shopping to feel ill. If you're feeling frustrated at having nothing to do, just you wait until after Christmas. You'll be busy from morning till night sorting out the stomachs and livers of the greedy souls who've eaten and drunk far too much and aren't prepared to pay the price without a moan and a groan.'

I assured her that I didn't in the least mind having a few peaceful days and hurried off into town to do some shopping of my own. As I struggled through the crowds and into a big store I couldn't help thinking what a difference children make to Christmas. Without them the festivities are in many ways a commercial hoax. Everyone buys cards for people he sees each day and presents for people he can't stand. But the smiles of children who have seen Father Christmas or who have spotted a toy they hope to get on Christmas morning are unforgettable.

I was lost in a quiet world of my own when the crush of

people in which I was immersed suddenly swept forwards. There were cries of 'Ooh!' and 'Ah!' and 'Watch out there.' Suddenly there came a shout from a few yards ahead of us. 'Get help! Someone's fainted.'

This was immediately taken up by others all around until everyone in the store seemed to be shouting 'Help.' Panic was only a few moments away when from within the Father Christmas Grotto came a red-coated figure with a flowing white beard. He disappeared beneath the sea of bobbing heads and I made my way as quickly as I could to the place where I'd last seen him.

When I'd finally managed to fight my way through I found the patient sitting up and taking big breaths. Father Christmas had one arm behind her and with the other he waved a thick Christmas number of a monthly magazine. The draught of cool air felt most refreshing.

'I'm a doctor,' I muttered to Father Christmas. I felt like a small boy again, hoping perhaps for a brand-new stethoscope or a black plastic patella-hammer. Unfortunately the effect was slightly spoilt by the fact that his white cotton-wool beard had slipped a little, to reveal a straggly and nicotine-stained handle-bar moustache.

'I'm the shop's safety officer,' he whispered confidentially.

'I'm feeling better now,' said the patient. 'I don't know what came over me,' she sighed.

'Probably the heat,' said Father Christmas.

'Very stuffy in here,' I agreed. We both ignored the fact that, if her sigh had been distilled, it would have retailed at several pounds a bottle.

Father Christmas went back to his grotto and I went back to my shopping.

Apart from the inevitable embarrassment when fifteen of the sixteen guests discovered, after discussing the ways in which they had managed to keep their earnings from the sticky clutches of the local tax inspector, that the sixteenth guest was the local tax inspector, the undertaker's party was a great success.

As we walked home Margaret and I held hands.

'Aren't the stars bright?' she said.

'Isn't Christmas a wonderful tradition?' I said.

'There's one star over there that seems much brighter than all the rest.'

'Traditions are the structure upon which the whole fabric of family life is woven,' I went on, pompous with the seasonal spirit.

'It's been a wonderful year.'

'It has, hasn't it?'

'Marriage is a wonderful thing.'

I nodded.

'Life's much more fun with someone to share things with,' said Margaret.

'And two can live as cheaply as one, as long as one of the two doesn't eat too much.'

'Or three.'

'Pardon?'

'Or three,' she repeated. 'Three can live nearly as cheaply as two.'

'Three?'

She nodded.

'Are you sure?'

She nodded again.

The stars in the sky had never shone so brightly and no Christmas was ever more beautiful.